ESSENTIALS OF MEDICAL VIROLOGY

Robert Wm. Pumper, B.A., M.Sc., Ph.D.

Professor of Microbiology,
School of Basic Medical Sciences of the
College of Medicine,
University of Illinois,
Chicago

Herbert M. Yamashiroya, B.A., M.Sc., Ph.D.

Assistant Professor of Pathology in Microbiology,
Abraham Lincoln School of Medicine of the
College of Medicine,
University of Illinois;
Head, Clinical Virology Section,
University of Illinois Hospital Laboratory,
Chicago

W. B. SAUNDERS COMPANY   **1975**
Philadelphia, London, Toronto

W. B. Saunders Company: West Washington Square
                           Philadelphia, Pa. 19105

                           12 Dyott Street
                           London, WC1A 1DB

                           833 Oxford Street
                           Toronto, Ontario
                           M8Z 5T9, Canada

Cover photograph: Electron micrograph of a thin
section of salivary gland virus infected mouse
tissue. Magnification 5000X. Courtesy
Drs. N. Grand and C. Joseph.

Essentials of
Medical Virology   ISBN 0-7216-7406-2

Last digit is the print number: 9 8 7 6 5 4 3 2 1

To our parents and families.

PREFACE

We live in an era when most of mankind's prominent diseases caused by bacteria have been dramatically reduced, and in certain cases eradicated, by vaccination, chemotherapy and sanitation. Laboratory techniques have become standardized for nearly all bacterial diseases and are performed at reasonable cost and with reasonable speed at most hospitals. Despite these facts, bacteria are still the major cause of death from infectious disease in the United States.

Viral diseases, on the other hand, have been prevented and controlled primarily by vaccination. Chemotherapy for viruses is in its infancy, and its efficacy is still questionable. Virus isolation techniques are at present complex, costly, time consuming and not yet even available at most hospitals. In clinical practice it is the physician alone who must often make the decision, on the basis of physical signs and symptoms, as to the possible presence of a viral disease. This decision may or may not be later corroborated by laboratory data. It is therefore essential that medical practitioners and health scientists be aware of the clinical features, epidemiology, risk, sequelae and control of all prominent viral diseases, as well as laboratory tests that are available for confirmation of specific viral involvement.

This book is a compilation of material pre-
sented in the virology portion of a didactic
course in medical microbiology to freshmen and
sophomore medical students. It is designed to
provide a quick reference to information on
basic and clinical aspects of human viral
disease for student and graduate health pro-
fessionals.

Robert W. Pumper

Herbert M. Yamashiroya

ACKNOWLEDGMENT____

The authors are indebted to Drs. Murray Batt, James Fenters, Samuel Nerenberg, and Ms. Roberta Smith for their editorial and factual comments during the course of the preparation of this book.

We also extend our thanks to Mrs. Virginia Ault for the typing of the manuscript.

CONTENTS ▬▬▬▬

Adenoviruses (Continued)

Chapter IX.

Cytomegalovirus (Salivary Gland Virus)

Chapter X.

Herpes Simplex Virus (Herpesvirus Hominis)

Chapter XI.

Infectious Mononucleosis

Chapter XII.

Varicella (Chickenpox), Herpes Zoster (Shingles)

Chapter XIII.

Warts (Verruca)

Chapter XIV.

Molluscum Contagiosum

Chapter XV.

Smallpox (Variola Major)

Smallpox (Variola Major) (Continued)

PART THREE   *RNA Viruses*

Chapter XVI.

Lymphocytic Choriomeningitis

Chapter XVII.

Coronavirus

Chapter XVIII.

Influenza

Respiratory Syncytial Virus (Continued)

Chapter XXIII.

Coxsackieviruses

Chapter XXIV.

Echoviruses (E.C.H.O.)

Chapter XXV.

Polioviruses

<u>Viral Hepatitis (Serum Hepatitis, Infectious
   Hepatitis</u> (Continued)

Chapter XXXIII.

<u>Miscellaneous Diseases</u>

Appendix:

Part One

GENERAL CONCEPTS OF VIROLOGY

Chapter I

GENERAL PROPERTIES OF VIRUSES

A. SIZE, MORPHOLOGY AND STRUCTURE.
   1. _Methods of study_.
      a. <u>Electron Microscopy</u>. Most viruses
are beyond the limits of resolution of the
light microscope and require special equipment
for their visualization. The electron microscope, with a resolving power of 0.01 mµ (1 mµ
equals 0.001 millimeter), is often used to determine size and structure. One technique consists
of shadow-casting by placing virus particles on
a metal grid and spraying them obliquely with a
sublimated metal. This makes them electron
dense, and when an electron beam focused by
magnets is passed through the specimen, and a
photographic print made, they have a three-dimen-
sional appearance. Another method, called negative staining, allows more detail to be seen and
consists of mixing the virus with phosphotungstic
acid (PTA). Subsequent photomicrographs show
surface detail of viruses due to the background
staining and penetration of spaces between virus
structural units by PTA. The virus, being less
electron dense than PTA, is "negatively stained."
      b. <u>Miscellaneous</u>. Filtration, ultracen-
trifugation and buoyant density have been used
to determine virus size. However, electron microscopy has largely replaced these methods.
   2. _Size_. Viruses range in size from 18 to
300 nanometers. One nanometer is equal to 10^{-9}
meter and is equal in value to 1 millimicron (mµ).
Size is often given in Angstrom ($\overset{\circ}{A}$) units, one
$\overset{\circ}{A}$ being equal to 0.1 nm. By way of review,
1 micron (µ) equals 10^{-4} centimeter or 10^{-6} meter.
As would be expected, there is a fair amount of
variation in size within a given species of virus.
This may be as great as 25 percent and is the

result of the variation in size *per se* combined
with inaccuracy of measurement. The smallest
virions are in the Picornavirus group (18 to
30 nm), whereas the largest are found in the
Poxvirus, Paramyxovirus and Rhabdovirus groups
(100 to 300 nm). Most other animal viruses lie
within a range of 40 to 120 nm.

    3. Structural Sequence and Terminology. The
genetic material of viruses is either ribonucleic
acid (RNA) or deoxyribonucleic acid (DNA), never
both. It is enclosed by a protein coat referred
to as a *capsid*. The capsid in turn is composed
of morphological sub-units called *capsomeres*.
These in turn are made up of individual protein
molecules called *structural units*. In certain
cases the capsid may be surrounded by a lipoprotein coat called an *envelope*. The nucleic acid
core and capsid together are spoken of as the
nucleocapsid. Some viruses have surface projections embedded in the envelope which confer
special properties on the organism. Two examples
are the hemagglutinin and neuraminidase projections
of influenza virus. The complete infective particle is referred to as a *virion*. A schematic
drawing of an enveloped virion is shown in
Figure 1.

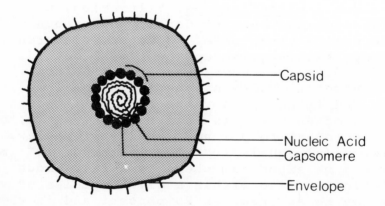

FIGURE 1. Schematic drawing of a virion.

4. *Morphology*.
     a. Cubic. These animal viruses have
capsomeres arranged in an icosahedral shape.
An icosahedron has 20 faces, each an equilater-
al triangle. The number and shape of the capsomeres making up the capsid is a characteristic of the particular virus group. Certain of
the cubic viruses, *e.g.*, herpes viruses, are
enveloped.
     b. Helical (coiled). The capsomeres of
these viruses are wound in a "spiral staircase"
manner around an extended nucleic acid core.
The helix may be wound into a ball and enclosed
in an envelope as is the case with influenza
virus.
     c. Complex. Members of the poxvirus
group, because of the nature of their structure,
cannot clearly be placed in either of the above
classifications and are spoken of as having a
complex morphology.
     d. Unknown. The capsid symmetry of sev-
eral groups of viruses has not been sufficiently
characterized to place them in any of the above
categories, *e.g.*, arena and oncorna viruses.

B. CHEMICAL CONSTITUENTS OF VIRUSES.
     1. *Structural proteins.* Viral capsid pro-
teins serve to protect the viability of the nucleic acid, especially during extracellular
periods, and to maintain virus structure. They
are responsible for the antigenicity of the
virion, and their antigenic mosaic is specific
for each species of virus. Attachment to a susceptible host cell surface is another property
of viral protein. Some viruses have as few as
two different proteins, others as many as 30.
     2. *Enzymes*. Unlike chlamydia and bacteria,
viruses do not possess metabolic enzymes, and
the number of enzymes that they do contain is
small. Ortho- and paramyxoviruses contain an
enzyme, neuraminidase, which can be visualized
by electron microscopy as "spikes" on the surface of the virus particle. This enzyme

functions in the release of virions from infected
cells. Its exact role in replication is not
known. Other virions may contain RNA polymerase,
nuclease or reverse transcriptase. Viruses may
also absorb enzymes from the host cell during
passage through the membrane, as for example
adenosine triphosphatase in the envelope of herpes virus.

    3. _Lipids_. Studies on the chemical content
of viruses have shown that a number contain various amounts of lipid. This content is well correlated with the presence of an envelope, and
structural units consist of glycolipids, neutral
lipids and phospholipids. The lipid composition
is the same as the membrane of the host cell in
which the virus was grown. Thus, the same species of enveloped viruses may have different com-
plements of lipids, depending upon the host cell
in which the virus was grown. All other properties of the virus species remain identical.
Lipid-containing viruses are generally sensitive
to inactivation by lipid solvents such as ether,
chloroform and desoxycholate. The exception is
the poxvirus group. It can readily be seen that
lipid solvent sensitivity can be used as an aid
in classifying viruses. The envelope serves to
protect the virion from extracellular inactivation.

    4. _Nucleic Acids_. Animal viruses have as
their genetic core either RNA or DNA and may be
classified into two large groups on this basis.
The property of infectivity lies solely in the
nucleic acid. This can be proved by extracting
the nucleic acid and showing that it has the
ability to produce complete virions. The infectivity of "naked" viral nucleic acid has been
shown with members of the RNA (picorna, arbo) and
DNA (papova, adeno) virus groups. The isolated
nucleic acid is much less infective than the
protein coated particle, no doubt owing to its
greater susceptibility to nucleases. Another
property of isolated nucleic acid is its ability
to penetrate and replicate in species of cells
which cannot be infected by complete virus. This
ability is probably due to removal of the capsid-

host cell receptor specificity. As would be expected, naked nucleic acid is not neutralized
by specific viral antibody directed against the
capsid protein. The nucleic acid may be double
or single stranded, and depending upon the virus
group, makes up from 2 to 25 percent of the total
virion. The nucleic acid type and strandedness
can be determined by a combination of RNA or DNA
enzyme susceptibility tests and acridine orange
staining.

C. CULTIVATION.
    1. _Methods_. All animal viruses require
living cells in which to replicate. This necessitates the use of one of the following three
substrates.
        a. Animals. Inoculation may be by the
intranasal, intraperitoneal, intracranial or
intradermal route. Most viruses are quite limited in the species of animal they can infect.
The determination of virus presence may be by
death of the animal or by skin, physical or organ
reaction coupled with pathologic and laboratory
diagnostic techniques. Diagnosis will be covered
under specific disease.
        b. Chick Embryos. Embryonated chicken
eggs (7 to 14 days old) represent a commonly used
substrate for virus growth. Inoculation may be
by the chorioallantoic, amniotic fluid or yolk
sac route. In certain cases the chorioallantoic
membrane may be exposed and inoculation carried
out by depositing the virus directly upon it.
Indications of the presence of virus may be
embryo death, pocks on the membrane, specific
alterations in the membrane cells (inclusion
bodies) or detection of virus in the embryo
fluids (_e.g._, hemagglutinin production).
        c. Tissue Culture. It is now possible,
by a relatively simple technique, to grow nearly
all human or animal tissues _in vitro_. Cultures
of this nature may be started from the tissue
per se, or purchased from commercial suppliers
or the American Type Culture Collection. The
latter organization maintains a stock of nearly

100 types of cultures from 20 different animal
species. Cells cultivated in this manner are
grown in sterile glass or plastic containers.
They attach firmly to the container surface
and, since they are normally one cell in thick-
ness, are called monolayers. In most cases the
cells are grown with a fluid overlay, but in
special instances they may be grown in or under
agar. The growth nutrient consists of a complex
mixture of amino acids, vitamins, trace metals,
salts, 5 to 10 percent serum, and phenol red as
a pH indicator. The virus specimen is deposited
directly on the monolayer or into the overlay
fluid. Many viruses have the ability to alter
or destroy cells during their replicative cycle
(cytopathic effect). Focal cell destruction may
result in the formation of plaques (holes) in
the cell sheet produced as the virus spreads
from cell to cell in the area of the original
infection. The microscopic nature of the plaque
(size, periphery, ballooning of cells, etc.) may
be specific for a given virus. Thus, plaque
formation is used as an aid to virus identification. Other indications of virus presence are
viral interference, inclusion body formation,
hemagglutination (ability of certain viruses to
attach to red blood cells) and serological tests
on the fluid overlay. Tissue culture has almost
completely replaced the use of animal and chick
embryo techniques for virus isolation.

D.   REPLICATION.
    1. *Growth Cycle*.
        a. <u>Attachment</u>. The first stage of viral
replication is adsorption to the cell. Viruses
attach through species specific receptor sites.
In some cases these sites can be shown to be cell
surface mucopolysaccharides.
        b. <u>Penetration</u>. The second stage involve
entrance of the virion into the cell cytoplasm.
Many viruses enter by means of engulfment by the
cell membrane (viropexis), and appear in the
cytoplasm in phagocytic vacuoles. Enveloped
viruses penetrate by fusion of the envelope with

the cell membrane.

     c.   Uncoating. The third stage, uncoat-
ing, involves the removal of the viral protein
coat. The exact nature of this step is not
well understood, but in all probability lysoso-
mal and cytoplasmic enzymes are involved. In
certain cases, as with vaccinia virus, a special
"uncoating" protein is synthesized following
penetration.

     d.   Eclipse. This period designates the
time between uncoating, when it is difficult to
demonstrate infectious virus, and the time when
mature infectious virus can again be detected.

     e.   Synthesis. This stage involves the
time in which viral proteins and nucleic acids
are produced in the cell.

     f.   Maturation. The assembly of viral
components takes place during this stage. The
nature of the maturation process is not well
known. It takes place over a period of hours
and in aborted infections frequently results in
the formation of "incomplete" particles, *i.e.*,
particles which either lack nucleic acid or
remain uncoated.

     g.   Release. Virions leave the cell by
slow release over a period of time called
"budding" or in one burst by cell lysis.

E.   INCLUSION BODIES.
  1. *Characteristics*.
     a.   Formation. Inclusion bodies repre-
sent cytopathic alterations which occur following viral infection. They are detected microscopically following staining and may be acidophilic (eosinophilic) or basophilic. They
are composed of mature virus, viral material
being synthesized, or they represent a cell
response *per se* to viral infection. They are
not formed by all groups of viruses but may be
characteristic for the virus that produces them.
Viral inclusions may be found in the nucleus or
cytoplasm, or in both sites.

    b. <u>Diagnostic Value</u>. The presence or absence of inclusion bodies serves as an aid to virus diagnosis. The type and location are characteristic for a given virus. A classic example is the cytoplasmic inclusion (Negri body) seen in neurons infected with rabies virus. In most cases, supportive studies, such as serology, tissue culture or animal inoculation, are done before a definitive diagnosis is made. It is possible to couple a fluorescent label to antibody specific for a given virus, add this to inclusion body containing cells and examine the resulting complex with a fluorescent microscope. This technique adds a high degree of specificity to the viral nature of the inclusion bodies. Inclusion bodies will be considered separately, where applicable, under each specific disease.

F.   INTERFERON.
    1. *Characteristics*.
       a. <u>Production</u>. Interferon is an antiviral agent synthesized by living cells as a result of viral infection. It may also be induced by exposure of cells to non-viral agents such as bacterial endotoxins, polynucleotides, rickettsia or synthetic pyran copolymers. It may be induced in either the intact animal or tissue culture.
       b. <u>Chemistry</u>. Interferon is a protein with a molecular weight of 30 to 80,000, is stable at low pH (2.0) and is trypsin degradable. When induced by non-viral substances, it may be detected in a matter of hours, has then a molecular weight of about 80,000 and appears to have been preformed. Virus-induced interferon has a molecular weight of about 30,000 and requires a period of several hours for synthesis and release.
       c. <u>Specificity</u>. The activity of interferon is species specific for the cells in which it was produced. It protects the cells against a wide spectrum of viruses. Thus, it

is cell specific and virus non-specific.

   d. <u>Mechanism of Action</u>. Interferon has
no effect on the isolated virion and only functions during viral synthesis. The direct inhibition of viral replication is due to a second
anti-viral protein synthesized by the cell under
the influence of interferon. This protein,
referred to as translational inhibitory protein
(TIP), prevents the translation of viral RNA on
cellular ribosomes. Isolation and characteriza-
tion of TIP has not yet been accomplished.

   e. *In Vivo* Applications. As might be
expected, the wide variety of viruses against
which interferon is effective raised the possibility of its use in the prophylaxis of human
diseases. This could conceivably be accomplished by either parenteral inoculation of preformed
interferon or *in vivo* induction by the use of an
interferon inducer. There has been great difficulty in producing sufficient quantities of
relatively pure interferon, and in most cases the
inducing agents have proved to be either ineffi-
cient or toxic.

G. EFFECT OF PHYSICAL AND CHEMICAL AGENTS ON
  VIRUSES.
  1. *Physical Agents*.
   a. <u>Temperature</u>. Autoclaving (121°C,
15 minutes), as normally used for bacterial sterilization, inactivates all known viruses. Similarly, dry air sterilization (160° to 180°C, 1 hour)
and boiling are virucidal. Temperatures of 56°C,
30 minutes, inactivate most virus species. Exceptions will be noted under the particular disease.
Drying also inactivates most viruses, but two
notable exceptions are variola and lymphocytic
choriomeningitis. Freezing has a preservative
effect on virus viability, and temperatures ranging from zero to -195°C may be used. The period
of viability varies from months to years, depending on the virus species and the temperature.
Temperatures below -60°C are efficient for long
term preservation of nearly all viruses.

     b.   Radiation. Ultraviolet light, λ, β, α and X-rays inactivate viruses.

   2. *Chemical Agents*.

     a.   <u>Ether</u>. Ether is highly effective for inactivating enveloped viruses. It has very little effect on viruses which do not possess this structure. An exception to this rule is the poxvirus group. Ether sensitivity is used as an aid in classifying viruses.

     b.   <u>Detergents</u>. The surface active detergents (alkyl sulfates, anionic and quaternary ammonium compounds) possess virucidal properties. Quaternary ammonium compounds, for example, are known to inactivate most animal viruses, an exception being the picornaviruses.

     c.   <u>Formaldehyde and Phenol</u>. These chemicals may be employed in a concentration of 1 to 5 percent to effectively inactivate viruses.

     d.   <u>Alcohol</u>. Methyl or ethyl alcohol in a concentration of 70 percent is highly efficient for inactivating most viruses.

Chapter II

CLASSIFICATION OF ANIMAL VIRUSES

A. PHYSICO-CHEMICAL CLASSIFICATION. On the basis
of their nucleic acid type, the animal viruses
are broadly classified as RNA or DNA viruses.
Further subdivision into virus groups and subgroups is based on their basic physical and chemical properties, *i.e.*, size, morphology (capsid
symmetry, number of capsomeres, presence of
envelope), and sensitivity to ether and other
chemical agents, as discussed in the previous
chapter. At present, 14 major groups of animal
viruses are recognized: 9 RNA and 5 DNA virus
groups. Medically important members of each
group and subgroup together with their physical
and chemical characteristics are given below.

1. *Ribonucleic Acid-Containing Viruses*.

Virus Group	Physical & Chemical Properties	Subgroups, Types
Picornavirus (Pico = small, RNA virus)	20 to 30 nm (mµ)* size Cubic icosahedral symmetry (32 capsomeres) No envelope Ether resistant	1. Enterovirus (acid stable) a. Poliovirus: types 1, 2, 3 b. Coxsackie A: 23 types c. Coxsackie B: 6 types d. Echovirus:over 30 types 2. Rhinovirus (acid labile)--over 100 types
Reovirus (Respiratory-enteric-orphan-virus) Also Diplornavirus (Double-stranded RNA)	60 to 80 nm size Cubic icosahedral symmetry (92 capsomeres) No envelope Ether resistant	1. Reovirus: types 1, 2, 3 2. Colorado tick fever
Orthomyxovirus (Myxa = nasal mucous)	90 to 120 nm size Helical symmetry Enveloped Ether sensitive	1. Influenza virus: 3 types Type A: many strains Type B: several strains Type C: antigenically stable
Paramyxovirus	150 to 300 nm size Helical symmetry Enveloped Ether sensitive	1. Parainfluenza: types 1, 2, 3, 4 2. Measles 3. Mumps 4. Respiratory syncytial 5. Newcastle disease

*In the metric system, with the meter as the basic unit of length, the common term millimicron (mµ) is expressed as nanometer (nm).

1. Ribonucleic Acid-Containing Viruses (Continued).

Virus Group	Physical & Chemical Properties	Subgroups, Types
Rhabdovirus (Rhabdo = rod or bullet shaped)	70 x 175 nm size Helical symmetry Enveloped Ether sensitive	1. Rabies virus 2. Marburg virus (simian)
Coronavirus (Corona = crown or petal shaped)	70 to 120 nm size Helical symmetry Enveloped Ether sensitive	1. Coronavirus
Togavirus	35 to 40 nm size Cubic icosahedral symmetry (32 capsomeres) Enveloped Ether sensitive	1. Rubella 2. Group A arboviruses:** Eastern equine encephalitis (EEE) Western equine encephalitis (WEE) Venezuelan equine encephalitis (VEE) 3. Group B arboviruses:** St. Louis encephalitis (SLE) Dengue: 4 types Yellow fever viruses
Arenavirus (Arenaceus = sandy; electron dense RNA-containing granules)	50 to 150 nm size Capsid symmetry not known Enveloped Ether sensitive	1. Lymphocytic choriomeningitis (LCM) 2. Lassa 3. Tacaribe complex arboviruses (So. American hemorrhagic fevers)
Oncornavirus (Oncogenic RNA virus) Also Leukovirus	100 nm size Capsid symmetry not known Enveloped Ether sensitive	1. ???Human leukemia and sarcoma viruses***

**The arboviruses (arthropod-borne) represent a large ecologic group consisting of more than 250 viruses with diverse physical and chemical properties. They have been divided serologically into several groups on the basis of antigenic relationships. In the United States major arbovirus infections are associated with EEE, WEE, VEE, SLE, and the unclassified California encephalitis (CE) viruses. In addition to the mosquito-borne encephalitides cited above, the tick-borne Colorado tick fever virus (Diplornavirus) occurs in the United States.

***The oncornaviruses include the avian leukosis complex, Rous sarcoma, and murine and feline leukemia and sarcoma viruses. Whether human counterparts of these viruses exist has not been established; they are the object of intensive current investigations.

2. *Deoxyribonucleic Acid-Containing Viruses.*

Virus Group	Physical & Chemical Properties	Subgroups, Types

Herpesvirus	100 to 150 nm size
	Cubic icosahedral
	  symmetry (162 capso-
	  meres)
	Enveloped
	Ether sensitive
		1. Herpes simplex
		   (Herpesvirus
		   hominis): types
		   1 and 2
		2. Varicella/Zoster
		   (VZ)
		3. Cytomegalovirus
		   (CMV)
		4. Epstein-Barr virus
		   (EBV)
		5. B virus (simian)

Adenovirus	70 to 90 nm size
	Cubic icosahedral
	  symmetry (252 capso-
	  meres)
	No envelope
	Ether resistant
		1. Adenovirus--over
		   30 types

Papovavirus
(Papilloma-
Polyoma-
Vacuolating
Agent)
 	
Polyoma virus
(mouse)
Vacuolating agent =
  SV40 (simian virus)
	43 to 53 nm size
	Cubic icosahedral
	  symmetry (72 capso-
	  meres)
	No envelope
	Ether resistant
		1. Human papilloma
		   (wart)
		2. ? Progressive multi-
		   focal leukoencepha-
		   lopathy (PML)

Poxvirus	230 x 300 nm size
	Complex symmetry
	Complex envelope
	Ether resistant
		1. Vaccinia subgroup
		   a. Vaccinia
		   b. Cowpox
		   c. Variola (small-
		      pox)
		2. Paravaccinia (Orf)
		   subgroup
		3. Molluscum conta-
		   giosum

Parvovirus
(parvus = small)
 	
Also Picodnavirus
	18 to 22 nm size
	Cubic icosahedral
	  symmetry (32 capso-
	  meres)
	No envelope
	Ether resistant
		1. Adeno-associated
		   viruses--at least
		   4 types: no known
		   disease association.

   3. *Unclassified Viruses*. The list of
medically important human viruses should cate-
gorically expand as putative and new agents are
isolated and characterized. The following agents
have not been sufficiently characterized for inclusion in the foregoing taxonomic groups.
   a. Hepatitis A Virus (HAV). The agent
of infectious hepatitis (IH) or short incubation
"MS-1" hepatitis was visualized for the first
time in 1973 by a technique called "immune electron microscopy." The very small (27 nm) spherical, virus-like particle resembles the parvo-
viruses in size and appearance. Attempts to cultivate this agent in cell cultures have not been
successful. The agent has apparently been transmitted to a South American monkey, the marmoset.
   b. Hepatitis B Virus (HBV). Three mor-
phologic forms are associated with serum hepatitis (SH) or long incubation "MS-2" hepatitis:
a small spherical particle (20 nm), a filamentous
form, and a larger (42 nm) complex sphere (Dane
particle) consisting of an inner core and an
outer surface component. The surface component
of the Dane particle is antigenically similar to
the 20 nm particle. Detection of DNA polymerase
activity in Dane-particle-rich purified sera
indicates this complex sphere to be the virion
per se and is presumably a DNA virus. The agent
has not been cultivated *in vitro* but has been
successfully transmitted to the chimpanzee.
   c. Norwalk (Intestinal Flu) Agent. This
agent is similar in size and appearance to the
Hepatitis A agent and may be a parvovirus or
picornavirus. It is associated with a common
ailment referred to as an "acute infectious non-
bacterial gastroenteritis" or "intestinal flu."
To date efforts to isolate and grow this elusive
agent in cell cultures or laboratory animals
have failed.
   d. Slow Viruses. Viruses have been
implicated or suspected in the etiology of several chronic and progressively degenerative
neuropathies. Because of the extraordinarily long
incubation period (months to years) of the

neurologic disorders, the putative agents have
been referred to as "slow viruses." Viral etiology has been demonstrated in two unusual or
rare subacute spongiform encephalopathies:
Kuru, which was found only in the Fore tribe of
New Guinea, and Creutzfeldt-Jacob disease, a
pathologically similar neurologic disease associated with presenile dementia and of wider geographic occurrence. Attempts to visualize these
agents by electron microscopy have thus far been
unsuccessful. Both agents have been transmitted
to the chimpanzee and several other nonhuman primates but do not elicit any detectable antibody
response. They are highly resistant to heat,
formalin, and ultraviolet irradiation. These
properties are at variance with those of the
conventional RNA- or DNA-containing viruses.
Measles virus, a paramyxovirus, has been associated with a rare progressive disease termed subacute sclerosing panencephalitis (SSPE).

B.   CLINICAL CLASSIFICATION ON THE BASIS OF
     DISEASE SYNDROME. In contrast to physical
and chemical criteria, an exact biologic classification based on pathogenetic attributes of the
individual viruses is not possible. However, it
is useful from a clinical standpoint to medically
categorize the viruses according to their specific
involvement in various disease syndromes. It
should be evident that in such a classification
a given virus may be involved in the pathogenesis
of several clinically distinct diseases and that
similar clinical manifestations are associated
with unrelated viral agents. An individual's age,
health and immune status, as well as seasonal,
geographic and socioeconomic factors, are important variables which could influence morbidity
from viral infections. These important parameters
will be considered in greater detail in the ensuing
chapters on the individual viruses.
     Viruses implicated in a clinical syndrome are
grouped below according to their respiratory,
cutaneous, and central-nervous-system disease
manifestations and specific organ involvement.

1. *Respiratory*. There is considerable overlap between many of these viruses in their specific roles in upper and lower respiratory tract
illnesses.
        a. Orthomyxovirus Group. Influenza virus--
pneumonia, croup (children), upper respiratory
tract inflammations (rhinitis, pharyngitis, bronchitis).
        b. Paramyxovirus Group.
            1) Parainfluenza virus--croup, bron-
chiolitis, and pneumonia in children; upper respiratory tract illnesses in children and adults.
            2) Respiratory syncytial virus--
bronchiolitis, pneumonia, and croup in infants
and children; upper respiratory tract inflammations in children and adults.
            3) Rubeola (measles) virus--prodro-
mal catarrhal period; pneumonia (rare).
        c. Adenovirus Group. Adenovirus--upper
and lower respiratory tract disease in infants,
children, and military recruits, adeno-pharyngo-
conjunctival (APC) syndrome.
        d. Picornavirus Group.
            1) Coxsackie-Echo (Enteroviruses)--
upper respiratory tract infections; pneumonia in
infants (Coxsackie B).
            2) Rhinovirus--common cold and upper
respiratory tract inflammations; occasional lower
respiratory tract disease in children.
        e. Coronavirus Group. Coronavirus--upper
respiratory tract illnesses in adults.
        f. Herpesvirus Group.
            1) Cytomegalovirus--pneumonia in
compromised host.
            2) Varicella virus (*Herpesvirus
varicellae*)--pneumonia particularly in adults
(rare).
            3) Herpes simplex virus--tonsillo-
pharyngitis with vesicles or ulcers.
2. *Cutaneous*. Included in this group are
viruses which produce eruptions or rashes on the
skin (*exanthem*) or mucous membrane (*enanthem*).

The pathogenesis of many of these viruses involves upper respiratory tract infection with
associated lesions in the mouth and/or pharynx.

    a. Paramyxovirus Group. Rubeola
(measles) virus--maculopapular skin rash; vesicles (Koplik's spots) in mouth.

    b. Togavirus Group.

    1) Rubella (German measles) virus--
morbilliform ("resembling measles") maculopapular exanthem.

    2) Dengue fever (Arbovirus)--macu-
lopapular or scarlatiniform skin rash, hemorrhages in skin and mucosae.

    c. Picornavirus Group.

    1) Coxsackie virus--papules and
vesicles in pharyngeal area (herpangina); vesicular stomatitis with exanthem (hand, foot and
mouth disease); maculopapular rubelliform exanthem, mainly in children in "summer fevers."

    2) Echovirus--mainly maculopapular
rubelliform skin rash, occasional vesicular,
petechial exanthems in children; vesicular enan-
thems in mouth and pharynx.

    d. Herpesvirus Group.

    1) Herpes simplex virus--vesicular
lesions on the skin and mucous membrane, eczema
herpeticum (Kaposi's varicelliform eruption).

    2) Varicella-zoster virus--various
exanthematous stages of macules, papules, vesicles
and crusts in chickenpox (varicella). Unilateral
vesicular lesions on skin and mucous membrane
supplied by affected sensory nerves in shingles
(zoster).

    3) Cytomegalovirus--petechiae and
purpura ("purple patches") in cytomegalic inclusion disease (CID) in infants and children.

    e. Poxvirus Group.

    1) Variola (smallpox) virus--pro-
gressive lesions from macules to papules, vesicles,
and pustules. Hemorrhagic lesions in more serious
cases.

    2) Vaccinia virus--eczema vaccina-
tum as a complication in smallpox vaccinee or
contact; lesions resemble confluent smallpox;
generalized vaccinia (rare).

3) Molluscum contagiosum virus--
benign wart-like cutaneous tumors with central
umbilication.
     f. Papovavirus Group. Wart (papilloma)
virus--localized papular growths or plaque-like`
lesions (verrucae).
     Although most likely viral in origin, the
etiology of erythema infectiosum (fifth disease)
and roseola infantum (exanthema subitum, sixth
disease) has not been established. These acute
benign infectious diseases with maculopapular
eruptions affect primarily infants and children.
The terms "fifth disease" and "sixth disease"
refer to an old classification whereby measles,
scarlet fever, rubella and Duke's (rubella-like)
disease were designated first through fourth
diseases.
     3. *Central Nervous System*. Viral patho-
genesis of the central nervous system (CNS) is
manifested primarily in the aseptic meningitides,
encephalitides, and paralytic diseases. The
term "aseptic" is descriptive of the clear cerebrospinal fluid found in viral CNS infections,
indicating an abacterial, nonpurulent disease
process. An encephalitogenic complication of
several natural virus infections, particularly
measles, is referred to as postinfectious or post-
infection encephalitis. Postinfectious encephalitis is believed to represent a delayed hypersensitivity reaction which may also follow rabies
and smallpox vaccination (postvaccination encephalitis).
     a. Picornavirus Group.
     1) Poliovirus--paralytic polio-
myelitis, aseptic meningitis.
     2) Coxsackie virus--aseptic menin-
gitis, encephalitis, paralysis.
     3) Echovirus--aseptic meningitis,
encephalitis, paralysis.
     b. Paramyxovirus Group.
     1) Mumps virus--aseptic meningitis,
meningoencephalitis, paralytic polio-like syndrome, postinfectious encephalitis.
     2) Measles virus--postinfectious

encephalitis, subacute sclerosing panencephalitis
(SSPE).

    c.   Herpesvirus Group.

       1) Herpes simplex virus--aseptic
meningitis, meningoencephalitis, encephalitis.

       2) Varicella-zoster virus--post-
infectious encephalitis, post-varicella encephalopathy and fatty liver degeneration (Reye's
Syndrome), aseptic meningitis (rare), zoster
encephalomyelitis.

    d.   Togavirus Group.

       1) Group A arboviruses (EEE, WEE,
VEE)--encephalitis.

       2) Group B arboviruses (SLE)--
encephalitis.

       3) Unclassified California encepha-
litis virus*--encephalitis.

       4) Rubella virus--postinfectious
encephalitis, congenital encephalitic syndrome.

    e.   Rhabdovirus Group. Rabies virus--
progressive, general, flaccid paralysis, postvaccination encephalitis.

    f.   Arenavirus Group. Lymphocytic chorio-
meningitis virus--aseptic meningitis, encepha-
loymelitis (rare).

    g.   Orthomyxovirus Group. Influenza virus--
encephalitis (rare), post-influenza B encephalopathy and fatty liver degeneration (Reye's
syndrome).

    Viruses are also involved in the pathogenesis
of several rare chronic and progressively degenerative neurologic disorders. Slow viruses are
the cause of two unusual subacute spongiform encephalopathies: Kuru and Creutzfeldt-Jacob disease. Papovaviruses are associated with a rare
neuropathy designated progressive multifocal
leukoencephalopathy (PML). The Guillain-Barre
syndrome (polyradiculoneuritis) is suspected to
be viral in origin.

    4. *Eye, Ear and Salivary Gland.* Listed
below are those viruses most frequently involved
in eye, ear and salivary gland disease syndromes.
In many cases, the ocular and otic clinical

---

*The California encephalitis viruses are placed
 here for convenience only.

manifestations are part of a primary respiratory, cutaneous or neurologic disease syndrome.

    a. Adenovirus Group. Adenovirus--follicular conjunctivitis, keratoconjunctivitis, pharyngoconjunctival fever, hearing loss.

    b. Herpesvirus Group.

        1) Herpes simplex virus--keratitis, keratouveitis, blepharitis.

        2) Varicella-zoster virus--zoster ophthalmicus: conjunctivitis, keratitis, scleritis, iridocyclitis, optic neuritis, pupillary and oculomotor paralysis; zoster oticus.

        3) Cytomegalovirus--salivary gland virus disease; *congenital* chorioretinitis, cataracts, scleritis, uveitis, deafness.

    c. Paramyxovirus Group.

        1) Measles virus--prodromal mucopurulent conjunctivitis, punctate keratitis in severe disease.

        2) Mumps virus--parotitis; conjunctivitis, occasional episcleritis and keratitis, optic neuritis (papillitis); neurosensory deafness.

        3) Newcastle disease virus--mild conjunctivitis, palpebral edema.

    d. Togavirus Group. Rubella virus--catarrhal or follicular conjunctivitis, mild keratitis; *congential ocular rubella* (microphthalmos, iris hypoplasia, cataract); less commonly retinopathy, glaucoma, and strabismus; neurosensory hearing loss.

    e. Poxvirus Group.

        1) Variola virus--catarrhal conjunctivitis.

        2) Vaccinia virus--purulent conjunctivitis, keratitis, blepharoconjunctivitis.

        3) Molluscum contagiosum virus--palpebral tumors with secondary conjunctivitis and possible keratitis.

    f. Papovavirus Group. Wart virus--papilliform warts on eyelid, conjunctivitis, keratitis.

NOTE: The Chlamydiae which are no longer classified with the true viruses, include the medically important trachoma and inclusion conjunctivitis (TRIC) agents. Trachoma is a chronic
keratoconjunctivitis which sometimes leads to
blindness. Inclusion conjunctivitis presents
mainly as a transnatally acquired acute purulent
conjunctivitis of the newborn. In adults this
venereally transmitted infection may occasionally produce a follicular conjunctivitis following accidental contamination of the eyes.

   5. *Cardiovascular and Muscular*. Viruses,
particularly members of the Enterovirus group,
are increasingly being recognized as etiologic
agents of myositis and cardiovascular inflammation.

      a. Picornavirus Group (Enterovirus
subgroup)

         1) Coxsackie B virus--myocarditis,
pericarditis, pleurodynia (epidemic myalgia,
Bornholm disease).

         2) Coxsackie A virus--myocarditis
(less frequently), myalgia.

         3) Echovirus--myocarditis (less
frequently), myalgia.

      b. Orthomyxovirus Group. Influenza
virus--myalgia, acute benign pericarditis, possible myocarditis.

      c. Paramyxovirus Group.

         1) Mumps virus--myocarditis, peri-
carditis (less frequently), postnatal endo-
cardial fibroelastosis.

         2) Measles virus--myocarditis/peri-
carditis (rare).

      d. Togavirus Group.

         1) Rubella virus--neonatal myo-
carditis and myositis in congenital syndrome.

         2) Dengue fever--severe myalgia.

         3) Yellow fever--severe myalgia.

      e. Herpesvirus Group. Varicella virus--
pericarditis/myocarditis (rare).

   6. *Joint*.

      a. Togavirus Group.

      1)   Rubella virus--transient arth-
ralgia and arthritis, particularly in women.
      2)   Dengue fever virus--acute arth-
ralgia.
    b. <u>Paramyxovirus Group</u>. Mumps virus--
arthralgia and migratory polyarthritis.
    c. <u>Unclassified</u>. Hepatitis A and B
viruses--arthralgia and nonmigratory, symmetric
polyarthritis.
    7. *Gastrointestinal*. Gastrointestinal symp-
tomatology (diarrhea, vomiting, abdominal cramps)
may accompany infection with a number of viruses,
particularly members of the enterovirus subgroup
of picornaviruses. The recent discovery of the
Norwalk agent, presumably a picornavirus or parvovirus, further signifies the possible role of
viruses as etiologic agents of acute gastroenteritis.
    a. <u>Picornavirus Group</u>. Coxsackie-Echo-
viruses--diarrhea, gastroenteritis in infants
and children.
    b. <u>Unclassified</u>. Norwalk agent--gastro-
enteritis ("intestinal flu") affecting all age
groups.
    c. <u>Adenovirus Group</u>. Adenovirus--diar-
rhea, gastroenteritis in infants and children
(sporadic outbreaks).
    d. <u>Reovirus Group</u>. Reovirus--steator-
rheic diarrhea in children.
    8. *Urogenital*. Genital disorders involving
mumps and herpes simplex viruses are well recognized. Urogenital manifestations are a relatively uncommon clinical finding in other viral infections.
    a. <u>Paramyxovirus Group</u>. Mumps virus--
orchitis, epididymitis, ovaritis, prostatitis,
urethritis as a manifestation of mumps (parotitis).
    b. <u>Herpesvirus Group</u>.
      1)   Herpesvirus hominis (type 2)--
cervicitis, vulvovaginitis, penile herpes, urethritis; carcinoma of the cervix(?).
      2)   Cytomegalovirus--cervicitis.

3) Herpesvirus varicellae--orchitis accompanying chickenpox.

   c. Picornavirus Group.

1) Coxsackie B virus--orchitis associated with pleurodynia.

2) Coxsackie A virus--genital ulcerations accompanying herpangina.

   d. Papovavirus Group. Human wart virus--genital warts on glans penis or in urethral orifice.

   e. Adenovirus Group. Adenovirus--acute hemorrhagic cystitis.

9. *Hepatic*. Acute viral hepatitis is associated primarily with the agents of "infectious" (Type A) and "serum" (Type B) hepatitis. Hepatitis may also be caused by other viral agents which localize in the liver and produce hepatocellular damage. Splenomegaly frequently accompanies hepatic involvement as a visceral complication of lymphatic diseases (*e.g.*, infectious mononucleosis) and in disseminated viral diseases of the newborn.

   a. Unclassified Viruses.

1) Hepatitis A virus--"infectious" or "short-incubation" hepatitis primarily in children and young adults.

2) Hepatitis B virus--"serum" or "long-incubation" hepatitis affecting all age groups.

   b. Herpesvirus Group.

1) Cytomegalovirus--hepatosplenomegaly, jaundice, and hepatitis in congenital cytomegalic inclusion disease; chronic hepatitis in acquired infections.

2) Epstein-Barr virus--splenomegaly, hepatomegaly with or without jaundice in children and young adults with infectious mononucleosis.

3) Herpesvirus varicellae--hepatitis as a rare complication of adult chickenpox.

4) Herpes simplex virus--hepatic necrosis with jaundice, splenomegaly in generalized neonatal disease.

   c. Togavirus Group.

1) Rubella virus--hepatomegaly with

possible jaundice, splenomegaly, in congenital
disease syndrome.
         2)   Yellow fever virus--hepatic
necrosis and jaundice in severe disease.
       d.   Picornavirus Group. Coxsackie virus--
hepatitis in generalized disease of the newborn;
possible hepatitis in children and adults (rare).

Chapter III

ISOLATION AND IDENTIFICATION OF VIRUSES

A. VIRAL ISOLATION. The principal method for isolation of viruses from clinical material is the use of cell culture substrates. Certain fastidious viruses which do not grow or grow poorly in cell culture can be isolated in laboratory animal or chick embryo host systems, as described in Chapter I. However, cell cultures will support the replication of most of the medically important viruses.

Primary cells and cell strains share genetic and biologic properties similar to those of the parent tissue from which they are derived and are generally more sensitive substrates than cell lines for virus isolation. Because there is no one cell type in which all viruses will replicate, most diagnostic virology laboratories will employ a combination of cell cultures for viral isolation studies.

The cell cultures are usually maintained as peripheral sheets or monolayers in test tubes. Following inoculation of a clinical specimen, the cultures are incubated at 35° to 37°C and examined daily for microscopic evidence of viral multiplication. Three types of cultures are employed:

1. _Primary Cultures_. The first passage of cells or tissue *in vitro* is called a primary culture. This type of culture may be prepared from any human or lower-animal tissue. Human and monkey embryonic kidneys are commonly used because of the ease with which they may be grown *in vitro* and the wide spectrum of viruses to which they are susceptible. The surgically excised organ or tissue is minced by means of a scissors or forceps and the cells dispersed with a proteolytic enzyme such as trypsin. The cell suspension is placed in sterile glass or plastic flasks or tubes in a complex growth medium which

contains amino acids, vitamins and 10 percent
serum. Penicillin, streptomycin and fungizone
are usually added to retard bacterial and
mycotic contamination. Primary cultures consist of a mixture of cells which are common to
the organ or tissue of origin.

 2. _Diploid Cell Strains_. These cultures
consist of cells which can only be cultivated
for a finite period and thus have a limited
in vitro life span. The Wl-38 fibroblast cell
strain, derived from embryonic human lung
tissue, is an example of this type of culture.
These cells are available from commercial suppliers and are used extensively in virology.

 3. _Established Cell Lines_. Cultures of
this type consist of cells which have a hetero-
ploid karyotype and an indefinite (infinite?)
in vitro lifespan. Examples of this type of
culture are HeLa cells, derived from human
carcinoma of the cervix, and HEp #2, derived
from human carcinoma of the larynx. Cells of
both these lines have an epithelioid morphology.

B. DETECTION AND RECOGNITION OF VIRAL INFECTIONS.
Several criteria are employed for the detection
and recognition of viral infection in cell cultures. Employing the criteria outlined below,
the virology laboratory can provide the physician
with a presumptive identification of a viral
isolate with a high degree of accuracy.

 1. _Cytopathology_. During the course of viral
multiplication, characteristic alterations or
degenerative changes occur in the morphology of
the infected cells. The viral cytopathogenic
effect (CPE) may be manifested by focal or diffuse
rounding of cells, cytoplasmic vacuolation or
ballooning, nuclear pyknosis, and formation of
multinucleated giant cells (syncytia).

  a. Picornavirus Group. Rapid and extensive cell destruction is associated with enterovirus (polio, coxsackie, echo) growth with rounding, shrinkage and marked nuclear pyknosis of the

infected cells. The CPE of rhinoviruses is similar but less extensive and optimal viral multiplication occurs at a lower incubation temperature (33°C).

b. Paramyxovirus Group. Members of the
paramyxovirus group (respiratory syncytial,
mumps, measles, parainfluenza type 2) character-
istically produce multinucleated syncytial cells
during their growth. Syncytium formation results
from fusion of the infected cells. Syncytia
produced by RSV may consist of several hundred
nuclei. A "foamy" type of cytoplasmic degeneration occurs during measles virus replication.

c. Adenovirus Group. Adenovirus growth
is characterized by rounding and enlargement of
the infected cells and aggregation into "grape-
like" clusters.

d. Herpesvirus Group. Cell rounding and
swelling accompany growth of members of the herpesvirus group (herpes simplex, cytomegalovirus,
varicella-zoster). The CPE is usually rapid and
extensive with "ballooning" degeneration in HSV
infection, whereas the lesion is slow in development and focal in nature in CMV and V-Z infections.
Syncytia are formed during HSV (especially type 2)
and V-Z virus growth.

e. Poxvirus Group. Foci of rounded cells
which degenerate into clear plaques are found in
variola and vaccinia virus infections. Variola
virus produces hyperplastic proliferative foci
in certain malignant cell lines, such as HeLa.
Formation of giant cells may accompany variola
virus growth.

2. Inclusion Body Formation. Inclusion
bodies are often formed during the course of viral
multiplication. The inclusions either contain
viral particles or represent cellular reactions
to infection. The viral inclusions may be sit-
uated in the nucleus or cytoplasm, or both, and
when stained with hematoxylin and eosin (H&E)
or other suitable stains, have eosinophilic
(acidophilic) or basophilic staining properties.
Two types of intranuclear inclusions have been
described:

     a.   Types of Inclusion Bodies.
         1) Type A intranuclear inclusion.
Homogeneous eosinophilic body found in central
area of the nucleus and separated from the mar-
ginated chromatin by a clear area (halo).
         2) Type B intranuclear inclusion.
Central mass or multiple discrete bodies formed
by condensation of basophilic material. The
earlier lesions may be eosinophilic or basophilic (amphophilic).
     b. Inclusion-Forming Viruses.
1) Herpesvirus Group.
    a) Herpes simplex virus ⎫ Intranuclear,
                           ⎬ eosinophilic
    b) Varicella-zoster virus⎭ inclusion
                               (type A).
    c) Cytomegalovirus--intranuclear type A
inclusion; intracytoplasmic amphophilic lesion
adjacent to inclusion-bearing nucleus.
    2) Adenovirus Group. Adenovirus--intranuclear
early eosinophilic bodies (most serotypes) and
characteristic basophilic mass or crystals
(type B inclusions).
    3) Poxvirus Group.
    a) Variola (smallpox) virus⎫ Intracyto-
                              ⎪ plasmic,
                              ⎪ eosinophil-
                              ⎬ ic or baso-
    b) Vaccinia virus   ⎪ philic in-
                              ⎭ clusions.
    4) Paramyxovirus Group.
    a) Parainfluenza virus ⎫ Intracytoplasmic,
    b) Mumps virus   ⎬ eosinophilic
    c) Respiratory syncytial ⎭ inclusions.
         virus
    d) Measles virus--intranuclear (type A) and
intracytoplasmic, eosinophilic inclusions.
    5) Reovirus Group. Reovirus--intracytoplasmic,
eosinophilic inclusions.
    6) Rhabdovirus Group. Rabies virus--intracyto-
plasmic acidophilic matrix with basophilic granules (Negri body). The characteristic Negri body
is demonstrable with Seller's stain using impression smears taken directly from brain tissue of
infected animal.

3. *Production of Viral Hemagglutinins*. The
hemagglutinating property of viruses is demonstrable by the hemagglutination or hemadsorption
techniques. In the hemadsorption test, the red
blood cells adhere directly to the surface of
cells infected with certain hemagglutinating
viruses. The hemadsorption phenomenon is especially useful for detecting members of the orthomyxovirus and paramyxovirus groups.

    a.   Orthomyxovirus Group. Influenza
virus--hemagglutination and hemadsorption of
various mammalian and fowl erythrocytes.

  b.   Paramyxovirus Group.

    1)   Parainfluenza virus ⎫ Hemagglutination
                      ⎪ and hemadsorp-
    2)   Mumps virus   ⎬ tion of various
                      ⎪ mammalian and
    3)   Newcastle disease ⎭ fowl erythrocytes.
        virus

    4)   Measles virus--hemagglutination and
hemadsorption of monkey erythrocytes.
(No hemagglutinin has been demonstrated for res-
piratory syncytial virus.)

    c.   Togavirus Group.
        1)   Rubella virus--hemagglutination
and hemadsorption of chick hatchling (1 day old),
pigeon and goose erythrocytes.
        2)   Arboviruses--hemagglutination
of goose, chick hatchling and rooster erythrocytes;
hemadsorption of goose erythrocytes.

    d.   Reovirus Group. Reovirus--hemagglutin-
ation of human erythrocytes.

    e.   Picornavirus Group.

    1)   Coxsackie virus ⎫ A number of cox-
                      ⎪ sackie-echo en-
                      ⎪ teroviruses pref-
    2)   Echovirus   ⎬ erentially agglu-
                      ⎪ tinate human type O
                      ⎭ erythrocytes.

    f.   Poxvirus Group.

    1)   Variola virus ⎫ Hemagglutination
                      ⎬ and hemadsorption
    2)   Vaccinia virus ⎭ of chicken eryth-
                       rocytes.

  g. Adenovirus Group. Adenovirus--a number of serotypes capable of hemagglutinating rat
and/or rhesus monkey erythrocytes.
  4. *Cell Susceptibility Spectrum*. Certain
viruses can be separated on the basis of their
ability or inability to replicate and produce
discernible alterations in different cell culture substrates.
  5. *Interference Phenomenon*. Replication of
a noncytopathic virus can be detected with a cytopathic or hemagglutinating challenge virus. This
technique is used primarily for detection of
rubella virus growth *in vitro*. Presence of rubella in infected cells will interfere with superinfection by a challenge virus, *e.g.*, enterovirus
or paramyxovirus.
  6. *Physico-Chemical Properties*. Viral agents
may be differentiated on the basis of their in-
herent biologic properties, by the effects of heat,
acid, ether or chloroform treatments on their replication.

C. SEROLOGIC IDENTIFICATION OF VIRAL ISOLATES.
Serologic procedures are used to confirm identification of a viral isolate. The suspected agent
is identified on the basis of its antigenic properties by using antiserums containing antibody
directed against specific viruses or their serotypes. Serologic methods most commonly employed
for virus identification are:
  1. *Neutralization (Nt) Test*. This is based
on the capacity of specific neutralizing or protective antibody to render a virus noninfective.
Where multiple serotypes of a virus exist, *e.g.*,
Coxsackie, echoviruses and adenoviruses, the
Nt test serves as a valuable epidemiologic tool
for determining the specific type of virus involved
in a disease outbreak.
  2. *Hemagglutination-Inhibition (HI) or
Hemadsorption-Inhibition (HAdI) Test*. A hemagglutinating virus can be identified by the capacity
of specific antibody to inhibit viral agglutination
of red blood cells *per se* (HI) or viral hemad-

sorption in cell culture (HAdI).

　　3. *Fluorescent Antibody (FA) Technique*.
Viruses in infected cells can be identified by
direct or indirect immunofluorescence techniques.

　　　　a. Direct FA. The fluorescent indicator
(*e.g.*, fluorescein isothiocyanate) is conjugated
directly to viral antibody globulin. The infected cells are reacted with the fluorescent viral
antibody conjugate and examined under the fluorescent microscope. Presence of viral antigen
is indicated by specific fluorescence in the
infected cells.

　　　　b. Indirect FA. The infected cells may
be reacted with unlabeled viral antibody and the
viral antigen-antibody reaction visualized indir-
ectly by adding fluorescent antibody directed
against the globulin portion of the complex.
Since viral antisera are usually prepared in
animals, the fluorescent indicator commonly used
is anti-species (goat, sheep, rabbit, etc.)
globulin conjugated with fluorescein isothiocyanate.

　　4. *Complement-Fixation (CF) Test*. Viruses
or their antigenic components prepared from
infected cells can be tested by the CF technique
using specific antigen-antibody complexes.
Unbound complement, as in the case of nonspecific
antigen-antibody systems, is detected by an indicator hemolytic system consisting of sheep red
blood cells (SRBC) and SRBC antibody (hemolysin)
which lyses in the presence of complement. If
the viral antigen is specific for the antibody
in the test system, complement is "fixed" and
no lysis occurs in the indicator system.

D. DETECTION BY DIRECT EXAMINATION OF CLINICAL
MATERIAL. Tinctorial examination of desquamated
cells for distinctive viral cytopathology has
been used for many years in the presumptive
diagnosis of certain viral diseases, particularly
those with cutaneous manifestations. Table 1
lists those viral diseases where direct examination of clinical material by cytologic techniques
has been useful in confirming viral involvement
in a disease process.

The direct examination technique is especially useful from a public health standpoint for differentiation of smallpox *vs* chickenpox lesions. In variola, the skin lesions show presence of intracytoplasmic inclusions; syncytial cells are not found. In exfoliative cytology, the finding of cytomegalic cells in urine is pathognomonic of cytomegalovirus infection. However, since excretion of cytomegalic cells may be intermittent, this direct cytologic technique is less sensitive than virus isolation methods. Electron microscopic methods have also been used to a limited extent for direct visualization of the poxviruses, cytomegalovirus, paramyxoviruses and the human papilloma and wart virus in clinical material.

The specificity and scope of direct microscopic examination methods can be greatly enhanced by immunologic techniques, viz., the use of fluorescein or peroxidase labeled viral antibody for demonstration of viral antigen(s). Examination of brain impression smears by direct immunofluorescence is now the method of choice for laboratory diagnosis of rabies. Immunofluorescent methods have also been successfully used in the rapid diagnosis of certain respiratory infections (*e.g.*, influenza, respiratory syncytial virus, adenovirus) by direct examination of desquamated epithelial cells from the naso- or oropharynx. This area of rapid diagnosis of viral infections is still in its infancy and should gain wider application for selected viral infections as standardized reagents for performing these tests become generally available.

TABLE 1   Viral Detection by Direct Examination of Clinical Material

Viral Disease	Source of Specimen	Histologic Stain	Microscopic Findings
Herpes simplex Varicella }	Scraping from base of vesicular lesion	H&E* Papanicolaou Giemsa	Multinucleated giant cells with intra- nuclear acidophilic inclusions.
Variola Vaccinia }	Scraping from papular and vesi- cular lesion	H&E Papanicolaou Giemsa	Intracytoplasmic acidophilic inclu- sions (Guarnieri bodies).
Measles (pneumonia) }	Nasal mucous aspirate	H&E Papanicolaou Giemsa	Multinucleated giant cells (Warthin- Finkeldey cells).
Cytomegalic inclusion disease	Urine sediment in cytomegalo- virus infection	H&E Papanicolaou	Characteristic large cell with prominent intranuclear eosino- philic or amphophilic inclusions; intra- cytoplasmic baso- philic lesion.
Molluscum Contagiosum	Exudate from wart-like lesion	Lugol's io- dine or bril- liant cresyl blue	Typical intracyto- plasmic acidophilic inclusions (mollus- cum or Henderson- Patterson bodies).
Rabies	Impression smear of brain tissue	Seller's stain	Intracytoplasmic eos- inophilic inclusions with basophilic gran- ules (Negri bodies).

*Hematoxylin and eosin

SELECTION OF SPECIMENS

A. SELECTION OF SPECIMENS. Clinical and postmortem specimens for viral isolation are generally taken from the anatomic site involved in
the disease syndrome. Depending on the nature
and clinical course of the infection, sampling
of different sites may be required to demonstrate an agent that infects one area primarily
and then gives rise to symptomatology by secondary invasion of another area, as frequently
seen in enterovirus infections. An outline of
specimens desirable for virus isolation is
shown in Table 2 according to disease syndrome
categories.

TABLE 2   Specimens for Viral Isolation from Different Disease Syndromes

Disease Syndrome and Etiologic Agent	Specimens for Viral Isolation	
	Clinical	Postmortem
1. Respiratory		
Influenza	Throat swab, washings	Lung, bronchial scrapings
Parainfluenza	Throat swab	Lung, bronchial scrapings
Respiratory syncytial	Throat, nasopharyngeal (N/P) swab	Lung, bronchial scrapings
Adenovirus	Throat swab, washings	Lung, bronchial scrapings
Coxsackie, Echo	Throat swab, feces or rectal swab	Tissues with pathologic lesions, intestinal contents
Rhinovirus	Throat, N/P swab	
2. Skin and Mucous Membrane		
Measles (Rubeola)	Throat swab, urine, heparinized blood	Lung, brain tissue
Rubella	Throat swab, urine, heparinized blood	Fetal tissues in congenital rubella
Herpes simplex	Vesicle fluid, throat or genital swab	CNS, liver and lung tissue
Varicella-zoster	Vesicle fluid, throat swab	Lung, liver, spleen tissues
Variola-vaccinia	Vesicle fluid, crusts, throat swab	Lung, spleen tissues
Coxsackie, Echo	Throat, feces or rectal swab, vesicle fluid	Tissues with pathologic lesions, intestinal contents

(Table 2, continued)

Disease Syndrome and Etiologic Agent	Specimens for Viral Isolation	
	Clinical	Postmortem
3. Central Nervous System (CNS)		
Enterovirus	Cerebrospinal fluid (CSF), feces or rectal swab, throat swab	CNS tissues, intestinal contents
Herpes simplex	CSF, throat swab	CNS tissues
Mumps	CSF, throat swab, urine	CNS tissues
Measles	CSF, throat swab	CNS tissues
Arboviruses	CSF, whole blood	CNS tissues
Rabies	Saliva	CNS tissues, animal brain
Lymphocytic chorio-meningitis	CSF, whole blood	CNS, lung tissues
4. Gastrointestinal		
Coxsackie, Echo	Feces or rectal swab, throat swab	
Adenovirus	Feces or rectal swab, throat swab	
Reovirus	Feces or rectal swab, throat swab	
5. Urogenital		
Mumps	Throat swab, urine	
Adenovirus	Urine, throat swab	
Coxsackie	Urine, throat swab, feces or rectal swab	
Herpes simplex (Type 2)	Genital swab	
Cytomegalovirus	Urine, throat swab	
6. Cardiovascular		
Coxsackie, Echo	Feces or rectal, throat swab, pericardial fluid	Heart muscle
Influenza	Throat swab	Lung, heart tissues
Mumps	Throat swab, urine	
Rubella	Throat swab, urine, heparinized blood	Heart and other tissues with pathologic lesions in congenital syndrome

(Table 2, continued)

Disease Syndrome and Etiologic Agent	Specimens for Viral Isolation	
	Clinical	Postmortem
7. Ocular		
Herpes simplex	Conjunctival swab, scrapings	
Adenovirus	Conjunctival swab, scrapings	
Newcastle disease	Conjunctival swab, scrapings	
8. Hepatic		
Hepatitis B	Whole blood for hepatitis-B antigen and antibody determinations	
Cytomegalovirus	Throat swab, urine, heparinized blood	Liver, lung, intestinal tissues
Yellow fever	Whole blood	Liver tissue
9. Miscellaneous		
Dengue fever	Whole blood	
Infectious mononucleosis (EBV?)	Whole blood for heterophile and EBV serology	
Mono-like syndrome (CMV)	Throat swab, urine, heparinized blood	

B. COLLECTION AND HANDLING OF SPECIMENS. Clinical specimens should be taken early in the course of illness; if possible, within a few days after onset of symptoms. In most acute viral diseases, the putative agent is rarely demonstrable in specimens collected during the patient's recovery or convalescent stage. *CLINICAL AND POST-MORTEM SPECIMENS MUST BE DELIVERED TO THE VIROLOGY LABORATORY PROMPTLY AFTER COLLECTION.* If there is a short unavoidable delay, specimens may be temporarily placed in the refrigerator (4°C). Specimens collected after normal laboratory hours should be stored frozen in a dry ice box or preferably in a -70°C mechanical freezer located in the clinical laboratory. Since certain viruses, *e.g.*, cytomegalovirus, varicella-zoster, and respiratory syncytial viruses, vary in their stability under deleterious conditions (standing for long periods, freezing and thawing, etc.), clinical material suspected of containing these agents should be collected at times when the virology laboratory can immediately process the specimens. Submission of more than one specimen collected on successive days greatly enhances the possibility of demonstration of a viral agent.

The procedures employed in the collection and handling of virologic specimens are generally similar to that used in clinical bacteriology with certain modifications as outlined below:

1. *Swab Specimens (Throat, Nasopharyngeal, Rectal, Conjunctival, Genital, etc.).*
        a. Swab specimens are collected with sterile cotton-tipped applicators.
        b. Place swab in sterile tube containing collecting fluid or transport medium provided by the virology laboratory. The transport medium usually consists of a balanced salt solution containing a stabilizing substance, such as gelatin, bovine serum albumin, or fetal calf serum.

2. *Throat Washings.*
        a. Have patient gargle with 10 to 15 ml of sterile Hank's balanced salt solution or other suitable fluid medium.

b. Collect in sterile screw-cap jar.

3. *Sputum*--collect expectorant in sterile screw-cap jar.

4. *Feces*.

a. Have patient defecate into bedpan and transfer with tongue depressor approximately 10 gm portion into screw-cap jar or container with a tight lid.

Note: A rectal swab is an appropriate substitute when a stool specimen is not readily obtained, *e.g.*, pediatric patients.

b. Liquid stools are collected in bedpan and transferred to screw-cap jar.

5. *Urine*--have patient void 10 to 20 ml of midstream urine directly into sterile screw-cap jar or other suitable container fitted with a tight lid.

6. *Cerebrospinal Fluid*--collect under aseptic conditions and place in sterile test tube.

7. *Vesicle Fluid*.

a. Aspirate fluid with a tuberculin syringe fitted with a 26-gauge needle, *or* rupture vesicle and absorb escaping fluid with a cotton swab, rubbing the base of the vesicle at the same time.

b. Dispense aspirate or place cotton swab into tube containing transport medium.

8. *Pericardial and Other Body Fluids*--place in sterile tube as for cerebrospinal fluid.

9. *Blood*.

a. Whole blood--collect 10 ml of blood in sterile vacutainer tube. No anticoagulants should be used.

b. Heparinized--draw 10 ml of blood into syringe containing 0.1 ml of heparin (1000 units/ml) and place in sterile vacutainer tube.

10. *Biopsy Tissue*--place in sterile petri dish on top of gauze moistened with sterile saline solution, *or* place in tube or vial containing transport medium.

11. *Autopsy Specimens*.

a. Obtain specimens as soon as possible following death. Care should be exercised to prevent cross-contamination of specimens by use of separate sets of sterile instruments.

    b. Place sections of each organ into separate labeled containers containing transport medium. No fixative should be used.

Chapter IV

THE USE OF ACUTE AND CONVALESCENT SERUM IN VIRAL DIAGNOSIS

Indirect evidence of viral infection can be obtained by testing the patient's serum for antibody against the suspected agent(s) involved in the clinical disease. For serologic diagnosis, at least two, and occasionally more, blood specimens are required to demonstrate a rise or appearance of specific viral antibody during the course of a patient's illness and convalescence. An initial "acute" serum is obtained immediately after onset of illness, followed by a second serum collected usually 2 to 4 weeks later during the patient's recovery stage. In some cases serologic results may be the only corroborative laboratory evidence of infection, especially where a viral agent is not demonstrable by isolation techniques.

In the performance of viral serologic tests, paired acute and convalescent-phase serums from the patient are titrated simultaneously in order to demonstrate a significant (4-fold or greater) rise in antibody titer. Although an all-inclusive statement is not possible, viral antibodies usually appear within a few days after onset of illness, attain maximum or peak levels at about 2 to 4 weeks, and gradually decline or disappear in a variable time period. The CF antibodies are generally detectable during a relatively short period of a few months to a few years, whereas HI and Nt antibodies usually persist for a longer duration, in many cases for the lifetime of an individual.

The CF test is most widely employed in the serodiagnosis of viral infections. The complement-fixing antibodies generally have broad immunologic specificity and reactivity against various antigenic components of the virus, making the CF test especially useful in viral diagnostic screening studies. The CF test, as well as the

HI and IFA tests, are less time-consuming and expensive to perform than Nt tests. Where a large number of antigenically distinct serotypes of a virus exist, particularly the Coxsackie- and echoviruses, serologic tests for determination of type-specific viral antibody are not practical unless performed with a specific virus isolated from the patient, or possibly with a serotype prevalent in a disease outbreak. In cases where particular antigenic types of a virus are associated with a clinical disease (*e.g.*, Coxsackie B virus myocarditis), serologic tests can be conducted with selected viral antigens. For determination of the specific viral serotype involved in a clinical illness, it is more feasible to type a virus isolated from the patient.

A. BASIC SEROLOGIC METHODS.

1. *Complement-Fixation (CF) Test*. In the CF test, patient's serum is heat-inactivated ($56^{o}C$, 30 min) to destroy endogenous complement and serially diluted twofold, usually as an initial dilution of 1:8 (1:8, 1:16, 1:32, etc.). Viral antigen is added, and if specific for patient's antibody it forms antigen-antibody complexes capable of "fixing" or binding a standardized quantity of added complement. Presence of unbound complement is detected by an indicator system consisting of sheep red blood cells and its homologous antibody (hemolysin). Complement not bound by the viral antigen-antibody complex will react in the hemolytic system, causing lysis of the erythrocytes. Conversely, binding of complement by the viral antigen-antibody system is indicated by lack of hemolysis (positive complement fixation). The CF antibody titer is expressed as the highest dilution of patient's serum capable of fixing complement in the presence of homologous antigen.

2. *Hemagglutination-Inhibition (HI) Test*. The HI test measures the capacity of specific viral antibody to prevent or inhibit agglutination of red blood cells by a hemagglutinating

virus. Patient's serum is pretreated with various reagents (trypsin, periodate, kaolin, etc.)
to remove naturally occurring nonspecific inhib-
itors of viral hemagglutination. Doubling dilu-
tions of serum beginning at 1:8 or 1:10 are prepared and reacted with a standard quantity of
hemagglutinating virus. If HI antibody is
present, it will inhibit the virus from agglutinating the appropriate species of red blood
cells. The HI titer is expressed as the highest
dilution of patient's serum capable of inhibiting viral hemagglutination.

    3. *Neutralization (Nt) Test*. The Nt test
measures the capacity of neutralizing or protective antibody to render a virus noninfective.
Tests for Nt antibody are usually conducted in
cell culture, employing inhibition of viral CPE
as a visible endpoint. The viable embryonated
egg or animal host systems are also utilized
with prevention of virus clinico-pathologic manifestations as evidence of presence of neutralizing antibody. The highest dilution of patient's
serum capable of rendering a standard quantity
of infectious virus noninfective is considered
to be the neutralizing endpoint or titer.

    4. *Indirect Fluorescent Antibody (IFA) Test*.
In the indirect immunofluorescence procedure,
acetone or methanol fixed preparations of known
virus infected cells are utilized as substrates
for titration of viral antibody. The viral antigen-antibody reaction is visualized by addition
of fluorescent antibody directed against the
antibody portion of the complex. The fluorescent
indicator commonly used is anti-human globulin
prepared in a heterologous animal species (goat,
rabbit, sheep, etc.) and conjugated with fluorescein isothiocyanate (FITC). Immunoglobulin
class of the viral antibody can be determined
by employing anti-human IgG or IgM fluorescein
conjugates. The highest dilution of patient's
serum giving definite fluorescence of virus antigen in infected cells is considered to be the
immunofluorescent antibody titer.

B.   SPECIAL HEPATITIS B SEROLOGY. Although specific clinical laboratory procedures are not
available for Type A viral hepatitis, a variety
of serodiagnostic methods have been introduced
for the detection of Hepatitis-B antigen (Australia antigen, Hepatitis-Associated-Antigen),
an antigenic component of Hepatitis B virus.
The tests are listed in the order of their relative increasing sensitivity for detection of
Hepatitis-B antigen (HBAg) and antibody (anti-
HB) in blood.

   1. _Agar_ _Gel_ _Diffusion_ _(AGD)_. This technique consists of placing an antigen and antibody
solution in separate wells cut in a special agar
gel. The reactants diffuse out from the wells,
and if they are specific for each other, a line
of precipitate is formed where they meet. Either
the antigen or antibody may be the "known" portion of the test. In virology, this test was
one of the earliest used to detect the presence
of Hepatitis-B antigen (HBAg) in blood. It requires about 24 hours for completion, and when
used for HBAg detection, has a low sensitivity.

   2. _Counterimmunoelectrophoresis_ _(CIEP)_.
This test is a modification of the AGD technique.
It is also referred to as counterelectrophoresis
(CEP), immunoelectroosmophoresis (IEOP) or cross-
over electrophoresis. It consists of placing an
electric charge across agar gel plates prepared
as described for AGD. In an electrophoretic
field, the HBAg moves toward the anode, and the
antibody (anti-HB) toward the cathode. Results
are obtained in about 1 to 2 hours, and it is
about 10 times more sensitive than AGD. The
CIEP test is the most commonly used method for
the detection of HBAg. A variety of inexpensive
units, complete with reactants and prepared agar
plates, are available from commercial suppliers.

   3. _Complement_ _Fixation_ _(CF)_. Complement
fixation may be used for the detection of HBAg.
The technique is the same as described for basic
viral serology.

4. *Passive Hemagglutination (PHA)*. In the
PHA procedure, either HBAg or anti-HB is chem-
ically coupled to the surface of erythrocytes.
The antigen- or antibody-coated red blood cells
thus serve as an indicator of presence of homologous antibody or antigen in patient's serum by
the hemagglutination reaction. The HBAg or anti-
HB titer is expressed as the highest serial dilution of patient's serum exhibiting visible agglutination of the appropriately coated erythrocytes.
In a modification of the PHA procedure, HBAg can
be detected by its capacity to inhibit known HB
antibody from reacting with antigen-coated erythrocytes (passive hemagglutination-inhibition).
The PHA test has also been employed for serologic
assay of rhinoviruses and HSV types 1 and 2
viruses.

5. *Radioimmunoassay (RIA)*. Radioimmunoassay
procedures have been employed for the measurement of a variety of physiological and biological
substances. Recently, the solid-phase immunoassay, or modifications thereof, is finding increasing application in experimental and clinical
microbiology for the detection of viral antigens
and antibody. In the currently licensed Ausria
ll-l25 (Abbott Labs.) method for detection of
HBAg, unlabeled guinea pig HB antibody is coupled
to an insoluble polymer bead (solid phase) and
reacted with patient's serum. Formation of
specific HBAg-anti-HB complex is detected with
iodine-125 labeled human antibody directed against
HBAg. The use of solid-phase assays facilitates
processing of specimens for radioactive counting.
The RIA method is the most sensitive procedure
available for HBAg detection.

C. VIRAL SERODIAGNOSIS. Serologic tests usually
performed for individual viruses are given in
Tables 3, 4, 5, and 6. They are separated on the
basis of four broad disease categories and are
usually done as a battery of tests on the basis of
the disease syndrome. Those tests which are not
routinely available at the hospital laboratory

level are often done by a State Public Health
Laboratory or the Center for Disease Control,
Atlanta, Georgia.

TABLE 3   Serologic Tests for Viral Respiratory Disease

Viral Antigen	Serologic Test	Immunologic Reactivity
Influenza A, B, C		
Soluble (S) antigen	CF	Type-specific antibody against viral nucleo-capsid or soluble (S) antigen which is identical for all influenza viruses of a given type.
Viral (V) antigen*	CF or HI	Strain-specific antibody against viral (V) hemag-glutinin which is specific for different strains within each type.
Adenovirus	CF	Group-specific antibody against common antigen (hexon) shared by all adenovirus types.
Respiratory syncytial	CF	Type-specific antibody against common antigen shared by several strains.
Parainfluenza 1, 2, 3, 4	CF or HI	Homotypic and heterotypic antibody responses occur against different sero-types; cross-reactive anti-body against parainfluenza type 2 and mumps viruses.
Mycoplasma pneumoniae** (Eaton's agent)	CF	Species-specific antibody.
Psittacosis (Ornithosis)**	CF	Group-specific antibody against the psittacosis-lymphogranuloma venereum group (Chlamydiae).

---

*For determination of strain-specificity, recently isolated strains closely related antigenically to influenza viruses currently involved in a disease outbreak are used as viral antigens.

**These microbial agents, which are no longer considered to be viruses, are usually included in a respiratory disease antibody screen for the differential diagnosis of nonbacterial "atypical" pneumonias.

TABLE 4   Serologic Tests for Viral Central Nervous System Diseases

Viral Antigen	Serologic Test	Immunologic Reactivity
Polio 1, 2, 3	CF	Type-specific antibody against intact virus.
Coxsackie Echo	Nt test with viral isolate or antigenic types	Type-specific antibody.
Mumps (Single serotype)* **		
Soluble (S) antigen	CF	Antibody against soluble (S) ribonucleoprotein antigen.
Viral (V) antigen	CF (or HI)	Antibody against viral (V) hemagglutinin antigen.
Measles**	CF	High antibody titers in cerebrospinal fluid and blood of patients with SSPE.
Arboviruses		

Group A: EEE, WEE, VEE
  Group B: SLE
  California encephalitis
    group
	CF
	HI
		Group-specific antibody.

Lymphocytic choriomeningitis	CF	Type-specific antibody.

* CF tests for mumps V and S antibodies are done in parallel. A *presumptive* diagnosis can be made on the basis of elevated S antibody titer in initial blood specimen. *Confirmatory* sero-diagnosis is made by demonstration of rise in antibody titers in second specimen collected about 2 weeks later.

**These viruses are most commonly involved in other than CNS disease syndromes, but are considered in a differential diag-nosis of aseptic meningitis or encephalitis and therefore are included in this table.

TABLE 5   Serologic Tests for Viral Cutaneous Diseases

Viral Antigen	Serologic Test	Immunologic Reactivity
Rubella	HI*, CF, IFA	Type-specific antibody (single serotype). Rubella IgM IFA antibody in congenital syndrome.
Measles	CF or HI	Type-specific antibody (single) serotype).
Varicella-zoster	CF	Homotypic antibody against varicella and zoster viruses; possible cross-reactive antibody against herpes simplex virus.
Herpes simplex	CF	Cross-reactive antibody against HSV types 1 and 2; possible cross-reactivity with VZ virus.
Vaccinia-variola	CF or HI	Cross-reactive antibody against vaccinia-variola group.
Coxsackie Echo }	Nt test with virus isolated from patient	Type-specific antibody.

---

* The HI method is also used for determination of rubella immunity.

TABLE 6 Serologic Tests for Miscellaneous Viral Diseases

Viral Antigen	Serologic Tests*	Immunologic Reactivity
Cytomegalovirus	CF, IFA	Cross-reactive antibody to three possible serotypes. CMV IgM IFA antibody in congenital syndrome.
Epstein-Barr Virus	IFA or CF	Type-specific antibody which is distinct from heterophile antibody in infectious mononucleosis.
Coxsackie B1-6	Nt, CF	Homotypic and heterotypic antibody responses against Cox. B serotypes; possible cross-reactivity with Cox. Gp. A agents.

Hepatitis B

   Antigen (HBAg) determination--RIA, PHA, CIEP

   Antibody (anti-HB) determination--PHA, RIA

---

* CF, complement fixation; HI, hemagglutination inhibition; Nt, neutralization; IFA, indirect fluorescent antibody; RIA, radioimmunoassay; PHA, passive hemagglutination; CIEP, counterimmunoelectrophoresis.

Chapter V

COMPROMISED HOST INFECTIONS

A.   COMPROMISED HOST.   <u>General Definition</u>:
Individuals who are incapable of mustering normal defense mechanisms against endogenous or
exogenous microbial agents because of disease
or chemotherapy.

B.   CONDITIONS PREDISPOSING TO MICROBIAL INFEC-
TIONS.   Severe, and sometimes fatal, bacterial,
viral, fungal and protozoal infections can
occur from primary and secondary defects in
humoral and/or cellular immunity, or from therapeutic measures which impair the phagocytic
and lymphocytic (B- and T-cell) responses.
Outlined below is a list of diseases or conditions predisposing to increased or undue susceptibility to microbial infections.   Although
not all-inclusive, it should serve as a start-
ing point in recognizing the general conditions
and factors which can alter the host-parasite
relationship in favor of opportunistic microbial pathogens.   Viral diseases, as a complication in the compromised host, are frequently
associated with defects in cellular immunity.
   1.   *Primary Immune Deficiency Syndromes*.
       a.   Infantile X-linked agammaglobulinem-
ia--recurrent infections with pyogenic bacteria
(staphylococci, streptococci, pneumococci,
etc.); no increased susceptibility to common
viral diseases and childhood exanthems.
       b.   Transient hypogammaglobulinemia of
infancy--develop recurrent infections mainly
with pyogenic bacteria.
       c.   Thymic hypoplasia (DiGeorge's syn-
drome)--develop frequent viral, fungal or
Pneumocystis carinii infections.
       d.   Immunodeficiency with thrombocyto-
penia and eczema (Wiscott-Aldrich syndrome)--
develop frequent bacterial, viral or fungal
infections.

      e. Immunodeficiency with ataxia tel-
angiectasia--develop chronic bacterial infections.

      f. Severe combined immunodeficiency
(autosomal recessive)--develop frequent viral,
fungal or pneumocystis infections.

   2. *Diseases or Conditions Associated With
Secondary Immunoglobulin and/or Cellular Defects*.

      a. Predisposing disease states.

      1) Carcinoma, Hodgkin's disease,
sarcoidosis.

      2) Leukemia, lymphosarcoma, multi-
ple myeloma.

      3) Diabetes.

      4) Nephrotic syndrome, uremia.

      5) Connective tissue disorders.

      b. Predisposing conditions or factors.

      1) Eczema, burns.

      2) Malnutrition, starvation.

      3) Extremes in age, particularly
premature infants.

      4) Traumatic incidents.

   3. *Therapeutic Agents Associated With
Immunosuppression*.

      a. X-irradiation.

      b. Anti-inflammatory agents--cortico-
steroids.

      c. Cytotoxic or anti-neoplastic agents.

      1) Nitrogen mustard.

      2) Mercaptopurine.

      3) Azathioprine ("Imuran").

      4) Cyclophosphamide ("Cytoxan").

      d. Antibiotics--chloramphenicol.

      e. Anti-lymphocyte serum.

C. DIAGNOSIS.

   1. *Clinical*. The physician should be aware
of the unusual role of viruses (and of course
bacteria, fungi and protozoa) as disease agents
in the compromised host and should be familiar
with the conditions or factors which favor their
establishment. The problem is magnified in organ
transplantation and cancer patients undergoing
treatment with immunosuppressive or cytotoxic

drugs and corticosteroids.   Thus, renal transplantation patients on immunosuppressive therapy
often develop severe pneumonias and hepatitis
from cytomegalovirus infection and cutaneous
eruptions due to wart (papilloma), herpes simplex
or varicella-zoster viruses.   In children with
leukemia, measles virus may produce a severe and
fatal rubeola with giant cell pneumonia, and possibly a degenerative subacute sclerosing panencephalitis.   Patients with Hodgkin's disease,
whose major immunologic defect is anergy, show
an increased susceptibility to disseminated varicella-zoster infection.

    2.   *Virologic*.   Laboratory confirmation of
viral involvement consists of direct examination
of characteristic or suspicious cutaneous lesions
for viral cytopathology and viral isolation studies.   Serologic techniques, as might be expected,
apply when the humoral antibody response is not
impaired.   Specific virologic procedures used are
given under the individual viruses.

        a.   Viruses commonly involved:
           1)   Herpes simplex types 1 and 2.
           2)   Cytomegalovirus.
           3)   Varicella-zoster.
        b.   Viruses less commonly involved:
           1)   Measles.
           2)   Vaccinia.
           3)   Wart.

D.   TREATMENT.   Treatment methods where available
are given under the individual viral diseases.
Examples for viruses commonly involved in compromised host infections would be 5-iodo-2-deoxy-
uridine or cytosine arabinoside for herpes simplex
and cytomegalovirus, and zoster immune globulin
for varicella-zoster.

E.   PREVENTION.   In cases of organ transplant or
treatment for cancer (leukemia, etc.), prevention
depends upon shielding the patient from exposure
to infectious agents during the course of immunosuppressive or cytotoxic drug treatment.   This
may be accomplished by isolation of the patient

in a special "clean" room, or by screening attend-
ing personnel for microbial "carrier" states. As
might be expected, the former method is most practical and often used; the latter is less practical,
less efficient and more time-consuming. Since
cytomegalovirus, herpes simplex, and varicella-
zoster viruses are so ubiquitous, and have a tendency to be latent in the tissues, there is a
real question whether either of the above methods
is useful in preventing viral infections. However, it should be remembered that a large majority
of compromised host infections are due to bacteria
and physical attempts at their prevention should
parallel those for viruses.

Chapter VI

ANTIVIRAL CHEMOTHERAPY

A. SCREENING TESTS.
   1. *In Vitro Assay*. Most screening tests
are done in tissue culture. A common technique
is to grow a cell monolayer, infect it with the
test virus and overlay it with a soft agar.
Sterile paper discs about 1/4 inch in diameter
are saturated with different concentrations of
the test drug, placed on the agar, and the cells
incubated. The drug diffuses into the agar in
a prescribed area, and if it has antiviral properties the cells in the area surrounding the
disc will be protected from destruction by the
virus.
   2. *In Vivo Assay*. Compounds which show
promise are further screened using a species of
animal susceptible to the test virus. In this
case the drug may be given by any of a variety
of routes and time intervals prior to or following virus inoculation. The end point used to
determine protection may be survival, prevention
of organ pathology or antibody conversion.

B. KEY INHIBITION POINTS OF VIRAL REPLICATION.
   1. *Nucleic Acid Synthesis*. In certain
cases where the virus has a replicative intermediate it might be possible to affect viral
replication by specifically inhibiting the intermediate.
   2. *Protein Synthesis*. Indications are that
viral messenger RNA's are different from host
messenger RNA's. Thus, it might be possible to
selectively inhibit viral messenger RNA tran-
scription.
   3. *Adsorption*. The primary step in viral
replication is adsorption, and this would seem
to be a fundamental inhibition point. Inhibition
would be best attained by action on the virus
per se rather than on the host cell membrane
where it might be deleterious to the cell.

C. CHEMOTHERAPEUTIC ANTIVIRAL AGENTS IN CLINI-
CAL USE.

   1. *5-Iodo-2'-Deoxyuridine (IDU, IUDR, Idoxyuridine)*. This drug has been shown to be effective *in vitro* against the animal DNA viruses, particularly herpes, varicella, vaccinia and cyto-megalovirus. It has found its most frequent use clinically against herpes type 1 infections of the eye. In this case it is administered as a 0.1 percent solution instilled in the conjunc-tival sac. It has been used parenterally in a limited number of herpes encephalitis cases. IDU in dimethylsulfoxide has been used topically for the treatment of herpes zoster (shingles). Com-plete, infectious virus formation is prevented by incorporation of the drug into viral DNA, thus inhibiting maturation. Viral resistance to IDU appears to develop readily.

   2. *1-Methylisaten-3-Thiosemicarbazone (Methisazone)*. Thiosemicarbazones have been shown to be active *in vitro* against poxviruses, certain of the adeno-, reo- and echoviruses, influenza A, parainfluenza, herpes, rhinovirus, varicella and poliomyelitis type 1. The *in vivo* use has been limited principally to the preven-tion of smallpox in contacts of this disease. There have been a small number of clinical trials using this drug to treat complications of vac-cinia. It is given orally and has the disad-vantage of being an emetic. Methisazone does not interfere with cellular metabolism or viral DNA synthesis. It exerts its antiviral activity by preventing mature virus from forming owing to faulty production of viral antigens.

   3. *Amantadine Hydrochloride (Symmetrel)*. This drug, a symmetrical amine, has been shown to be effective against one virus only, influenza type A. It is not functional against influenza B, C or paramyxoviruses. Human volunteer studies, using amantadine following influenza A_2 given by the nasal or oral route, showed a significant reduction in the number of cases. It must be administered before or shortly after contact with the disease. It could find application in the

control of epidemics of influenza A. It is given
orally and dose-related side effects (insomnia,
ataxia, dizziness, nervousness) have been reported. Amantadine exerts its antiviral effect
by preventing penetration of the virus into the
host cell.

   4. *Cytosine Arabinoside (Cytarabine, Ara-C,
Cytosar)*. This pyrimidine analogue is antiviral
in vitro for DNA viruses (herpes, smallpox, varicella, vaccinia and cytomegalovirus). It is not
effective against adenovirus. It has been used
clinically in a manner and in situations similar
to those pertaining to IDU. Cytosine arabinoside
is more toxic than IDU, but herpes virus is more
sensitive to it, and viral resistance to cytarabine has not been reported. It exerts its effect
by inhibiting viral DNA synthesis. It is not
selective for viral DNA but also inhibits the
production of cellular DNA. Adenosine arabinoside (Ara-A) may be less toxic at therapeutic
levels.

Chapter VII

ONCOGENIC
(TUMOR-INDUCING) VIRUSES

No human metastatic neoplasm has as yet been shown to have an infectious etiology. It is true that verrucae and molluscum contagiosum viruses produce small benign tumors in humans, but they never metastasize. It has been postulated that herpes simplex type 2 plays a role in the induction of human cervical carcinoma; however, a direct cause and effect relationship has not been established (see Chapter X).

Where lower animals are concerned it is a different matter, and a large number of viruses have been shown to possess oncogenic potential. This property is most often demonstrated *in vivo*, but with some viruses it may also be observed *in vitro* in cell cultures (cell transformation). The latter case has proved most interesting, for through this technique it was discovered that following cell transformation the virus *per se* was no longer detectable by standard methods. The identification of the role of the virus had to be determined by showing the presence of viral RNA or DNA or new antigens in the transformed cells. If this is the case with human tumors, searching for viral activity by standard techniques would be fruitless. Some of the characteristics of transformed cells are: 1. they produce tumors in isogeneic animals, 2. they have chromosome aberrations, 3. they form colonies in soft agar, 4. they do not exhibit contact inhibition, 5. they may have new cellular antigens, 6. they have a random cell orientation, and 7. they have an infinite *in vitro* life span.

Not all oncogenic viruses have the ability to produce "natural" tumors in animals. Some require special conditions to be met (experimentally) before this property can be expressed. For example: certain viruses have been isolated from a host in which they produce spontaneous tumors, and they may be used to produce tumors experimentally in the same host. Other oncogenic viruses may or may not produce natural tumors in the host of origin, may or may not produce tumors experimentally in the host of origin, and may be used to produce tumors experimentally in other hosts. Thus, in certain situations there is a natural association between the virus and the tumor, and in others, man must initiate the relationship. The oncogenic viruses are classified on the same basis as other animal viruses (see Chapter II). They may be divided into two broad groups on the basis of their nucleic acid:

A.   ONCOGENIC RNA VIRUSES (ONCORNAVIRUSES).
   1. _Murine Leucosis_. Several strains which produce natural leukemias in mice and tumors experimentally in mice, hamsters and rats.
   2. _Murine Mammary Tumor_. This virus produces natural mammary tumors in mice and may be used to produce tumors experimentally in the same host.
   3. _Avian Leucosis_. Antigenically related viruses which produce natural lymphoblastosis, myeloblastosis or erythroblastosis in chickens, and viruses which produce natural sarcomas in chickens (Rous sarcoma).
   4. _Feline Leucosis_. A group of related viruses which can produce natural and experimentally induced leukemias in cats and natural sarcomas in cats.

B.   ONCOGENIC DNA VIRUSES.
   1. _Adenoviruses_. Bovine (type 3), avian, simian and human (types 3, 7, 11, 12, 14, 16, 18, 21 and 31) members have not been shown to produce natural tumors in the host of origin but produce solid tumors in newborn hamsters, rats and mice.
   2. _Papovaviruses_.
      a. _Polyoma_. This virus has not been shown to produce natural tumors, is often found as a latent infection of mice, and can be used experimentally to produce a wide variety of solid tumors in newborn mice, rats, hamsters, ferrets,

rabbits and guinea pigs.

      b.   Simian Vacuolating Virus (SV_{40}).
This virus has not been shown to produce natural tumors but may be used to experimentally produce tumors in newborn hamsters.

      c.   Papilloma.

      1)   Human--the wart virus produces natural or experimental benign tumors in man only.

      2)   Rabbit--this virus produces natural or experimental papillomas in rabbits only (Shope papilloma virus).

      3)   Bovine--this virus produces a natural or experimental papilloma in cows only.

      4)   Canine--this virus produces a natural papilloma in dogs only.

   3.   *Herpesviruses*.

      a.   Frog. This virus produces a natural or experimental renal carcinoma in frogs only (Lucké tumor virus).

      b.   Avian. This virus produces a natural or experimental lymphoma in chickens only (Marek's disease).

      c.   Rabbit. This virus has not been shown to produce a natural tumor but may be used to experimentally produce a lymphoma in rabbits.

      d.   Monkey. This virus has been shown to produce a natural and experimental lymphoma in monkeys.

   4.   *Poxviruses*.

      a.   Molluscum Contagiosum. This virus produces natural or experimental benign tumors in man only.

      b.   Yaba. This virus produces natural or experimental benign skin tumors in monkeys only.

      c.   Fibroma. A group of viruses which produce natural or experimental fibromas in squirrels, rabbits, and deer. Myxomatosis is a highly fatal natural or experimental virus disease of European rabbits.

Part Two

DNA VIRUSES

Chapter VIII

ADENOVIRUSES

A. PROPERTIES OF THE VIRUS. Adenoviruses contain DNA as their genetic material, are 60 to 90
nm in diameter, have a cubic icosahedral symmetry
and do not have an envelope. The adenoviruses
are the only so designated members of this major
virus group. Thirty-one antigenic types, identified by neutralization, have been isolated from
humans. In addition to the type-specific neutralizing antigen, there is a group-specific complement fixing antigen (hexon) shared by all adenovirus types. The 31 serotypes may be divided
into four subgroups on the basis of their ability
to agglutinate rhesus monkey or rat red blood
cells. They are resistant to ether and chloroform but are inactivated by a temperature of 56°C
for 30 min, UV light and formalin. They remain
viable for weeks at room temperature at a slightly
acid pH and are stable for years at -70°C.

B. HOST RESPONSE TO INFECTION. Adenoviruses are
generally associated with mild upper respiratory
illnesses but may produce lower respiratory disease and other inflammations. There are several
clinical syndromes associated with the adenoviruses.

   1. *Incubation Period, Signs and Symptoms*.
Acute respiratory disease (ARD) is seen predominantly in military recruits and is caused by
type 4, and occasionally types 3 or 7, adenoviruses. It usually presents as an influenza-
like disease with an incubation period of 5 to
6 days. The syndrome consists of fever (101-
103°F), headache, chills, and malaise which lasts
for 2 to 4 days. Complete recovery without sequelae normally takes place. In young children and
particularly infants, types 1, 2, 3, and 5 have
been occasionally implicated in cases of bronchiolitis and a possible fatal pneumonia. A syndrome

clinically resembling whooping cough (*pertussis-like syndrome*) has been associated with these serotypes.

   Pharyngoconjunctival fever is a condition which is similar to ARD, often with the additional complications of inflammation of the throat and tonsils, and conjunctivitis. The disease is most often caused by type 3 and occasionally by types 5, 7 or 21. The pharyngitis usually resolves in 4 to 5 days, but the conjunctivitis may persist for as long as three weeks. In either case there are no sequelae.

   Conjunctivitis may occur without the associated ARD. It is follicular in type and may involve one or both eyes. There is lacrimation and a serous exudate which may last for several weeks. The incubation period is 2 to 7 days and the disease is most commonly caused by types 3 or 7 and less often by types 2, 5, 6, 9, 10 or 19. The condition is self-resolving with no permanent vision impairment. *Epidemic keratoconjunctivitis* (shipyard eye) is a highly infectious eye infection caused primarily by adenovirus type 8, and occasionally other serotypes. The incubation period is 5 to 7 days and the disease is marked by a sudden onset with edema of the conjunctiva accompanied by a mononuclear cell exudate. The disease is unilateral at first, but becomes bilateral after a few days. A low-grade fever and a preauricular lymphadenopathy are present. The keratitis consists of small opacities (0.01 to 0.3mm) which may ulcerate. Lacrimation and photophobia are pronounced. The condition may persist for weeks or months but normally heals with no permanent sequelae.

   Hemorrhagic cystitis is an acute self-limiting disease seen occasionally in children and is characterized by polyurea, dysurea and hematuria. It has been associated with adenovirus 11.

   2. <u>Pathogenesis</u>. The virus reaches the susceptible tissue which may be pharynx or conjunctiva depending upon the adenovirus type. Multiplication takes place in these cells, but the virus seldom penetrates beyond the associated

lymph nodes. Thus, a viremia does not occur.
There is also an obvious multiplication of the
virus in the gastrointestinal tract, since in
many cases of ARD or pharyngoconjunctival fever
the virus may be isolated from stools.

   3. *Pathology*. Adenovirus diseases are
rarely fatal so the pathology is not well known.
In the few fatal non-bacterial pneumonia cases
in infants from which adenoviruses have been
isolated, the outstanding pathology was in the
epithelial cells of the alveolar and bronchial
walls. There was necrosis, and the cells had
enlarged nuclei and a central basophilic mass
surrounded by a halo.

   4. *Immune Response*. Complement fixing,
hemagglutination inhibiting and neutralizing
antibodies appear in the serum 4 to 8 days following onset and peak at about 2 weeks. Evidence indicates that they persist for years in
low titer. In the case of CF antibodies, which
are group-specific, a heterotypic secondary response with a rapid rise in antibody titer occurs
following a previous infection with any of the
adenovirus group. The HI and Nt tests are type
specific.

   5. *Prognosis*. The prognosis is excellent
in all forms of adenovirus infection. Superinfection with bacteria may be a problem in the
case of epidemic keratoconjunctivitis. There
have been a few rare instances where adenoviruses
have been associated with fatal pneumonia in
infants.

C. DIAGNOSIS.
   1. *Clinical*. It is impossible to diagnose
ARD clinically as being due to an adenovirus
because of the large number of other viruses which
cause a similar syndrome. In the case of pharyngoconjunctival fever, the combination of pharyngitis, conjunctivitis and fever is suggestive of
an adenovirus etiology. Epidemic keratoconjunctivitis is easily diagnosed during small outbreaks
or epidemics, based upon the clinical picture previously described. Exact diagnosis of etiology

in all cases depends upon laboratory results.

   2. *Laboratory*.

     a. <u>Isolation of the Virus</u>. There is no suitable laboratory animal for the isolation of adenoviruses, but they may be grown in a wide variety of cell cultures. The most commonly used are human embryonic kidney or lung (WI-38), HEp #2 or HeLa cells. Swabs from the infected tissue (pharyngeal, eye, or urine in the case of cystitis) are best taken during the acute stage of the disease and inoculated into cultures of these cells. The virus is cytopathic for the cells, and intranuclear basophilic inclusion bodies are produced. Specific identification is carried out by neutralization with type-specific antiserum.

     b. <u>Serology</u>. Serum collected early after onset of illness and 10 to 14 days later is used for serological diagnosis. The group specific complement fixation test is most often used to establish the cause as being due to a member of the adenovirus group. Neutralization of known adenovirus types in cell cultures by the patient's acute and convalescent serum may be used to determine the specific type of adenovirus involved. Hemagglutination inhibition is rarely used. A fourfold or greater increase in antibody titer between acute and convalescent serum is necessary for diagnosis.

D. TREATMENT. There is no specific treatment for adenovirus infections. Topical antibiotics are often used to prevent secondary bacterial infections in epidemic keratoconjunctivitis. Aside from this, treatment is supportive.

E. EPIDEMIOLOGY. Adenovirus ARD is spread person to person via the respiratory tract and accounts for about 4 percent of civilian respiratory disease. Its major incidence is among military recruits where it may account for more than 50 percent of respiratory infections. The disease is endemic throughout the year, with the

major incidence in winter. Pharyngoconjunctival
fever occurs in epidemics in school children and
is spread person to person. It has long been
suspected that it may be transmitted through
swimming pools, since the virus is known to survive for long periods in sewage and water and is
present in the stools of infected persons for
weeks. The respiratory tract is the portal of
entry. Conjunctivitis without the associated
pharyngitis is probably spread by the same method.
Epidemic keratoconjunctivitis was first reported
in the U.S.A. in 1941 when it appeared in indus-
trial plants and shipyards on the west coast and
later throughout the country. Irritation to the
eye, such as dust, dirt or traumatic insult,
seems to predispose to the infection which is
spread person to person or by fomites. It is
not uncommon to have a number of cases occur in
ophthalmologic practice. In this case it is
spread from one patient to another by improper
cleansing of instruments (e.g., tonometer). The
frequency of the presence of antibody to epidemic
keratoconjunctivitis (adenovirus type 8) in the
adult population in the U.S.A. is about 1 percent.
Man is the only reservoir of human adenoviruses,
and their distribution is worldwide. Types 1, 2,
5 and 6 have been isolated from surgically removed tonsils and adenoids in apparently healthy
individuals. It is possible that infection with
these types takes place early in life and the
virus remains latent in these tissues. The virus
cannot be isolated from intact healthy tissue.

F.   PREVENTION.
     1. *Active Immunization*. There are no licensed
adenovirus vaccines available in the U.S.A. An
inactivated virus vaccine for the prevention of
ARD has been tested in military recruits. It contained types 3, 4 and 7, and was shown to reduce
the number of cases by 85 percent.
     2. *Passive Protection*. Although theoretically
possible, passive protection is not practiced in
the case of adenoviruses.

G. CONTROL.   In the case of ARD, no control is
practical.   In pharyngoconjunctival fever and
conjunctivitis, isolation of suspected cases
and proper chlorination of swimming pool water
may be helpful.   Strict attention to sterilization of medical instruments used in eye examina-
tions as well as handwashing after contact with
patients is a helpful control measure for epidemic keratoconjunctivitis.

Chapter IX

CYTOMEGALOVIRUS
(SALIVARY GLAND VIRUS)

A. PROPERTIES OF THE VIRUS. Cytomegalovirus
contains DNA as its genetic material, is approximately 110 nm in size, has a cubic icosahedral
symmetry, possesses an envelope and is classified as a member of the herpesvirus group. The
cytomegaloviruses of man may be grouped on the
basis of related complement fixing antigens.
Minor strain differences may be detected by
neutralization. The virus is inactivated by
lipid solvents, such as ether or chloroform, and
by a temperature of 56 to 60°C for 30 minutes.
It retains its infectivity for months when stored
at -70 to -90°C in a 30 percent solution of sor-
bitol, and for longer periods when stored in a
liquid nitrogen refrigerator.

B. HOST RESPONSE TO INFECTION.
1. _Incubation Period, Signs and Symptoms_.
The incubation period is not known, but in those
instances where the virus has been shown to be
transmitted by transfusion of fresh whole blood
the incubation period has been found to be about
30 to 40 days.
a. Prenatal Infection. The virus may be
acquired as a congenital infection (congenital
cytomegalic inclusion disease) from a primary or
reactivated latent infection in the mother. As
a consequence, any of the following may result:
1) an asymptomatic infection with virus excreted
in the urine, 2) a condition where there is low
birth weight, microcephaly, chorioretinitis and
mental·retardation or motor disabilities, 3) a
condition which may show up years later as mental
retardation, or 4) a severe generalized infection
with a hemorrhagic tendency, petechiae, hepatosplenomegaly, jaundice and hemolytic anemia.
b. Mononucleosis. Cytomegalovirus mononucleosis is an acute febrile disease which may

follow the transfusion of large volumes of fresh
whole blood. It resembles infectious mononucleosis hematologically, but there is no exudative
tonsillopharyngitis or rise in heterophile antibody (see Chapter XI). Cytomegalovirus can be
isolated from peripheral lymphocytes of these
patients. Similar cases have been shown to occur
in the absence of blood transfusions.

      c. <u>Compromised Host</u>. Cytomegalovirus
infections present a special problem under these
conditions (see Chapter V). An interstitial
pneumonia and fever are common findings, and the
virus is usually disseminated throughout the body.

      2. *Pathology*. The characteristic altera-
tion seen by microscopic examination of infected
cells is increased cell size and the formation
of large (15 µ) spherical amphophilic nuclear
and smaller (2 to 4 µ) basophilic cytoplasmic
inclusion bodies, the typical so-called "owl
eye" inclusions. In the liver and other organs
there may be areas of focal necrosis and in the
brain necrotizing granulomatous lesions and
periventricular calcification. The organ pathology in congenital infections is the result of
destruction of formed tissue and not due to an
inhibition of organogenesis.

      3. *Immune Response*. Complement fixing and
neutralizing antibodies are produced as a result
of infection. Reinfection and virus excretion
can take place even though serum neutralizing
antibody is present. The effectiveness of transplacentally acquired maternal IgG in protecting
the neonate is not known, but in the light of
the previous statement, it would be expected to
be questionable. Following primary infection,
levels of CF and Nt antibodies are detectable for
several years. It is probable that reinfection
and viral latency reactivation play a role in
maintaining these levels.

      4. *Prognosis*. Most of the infections caused
by cytomegalovirus are subclinical and rarely result in medical problems. Severe generalized disease, which usually manifests itself clinically
in the first week of life, often has a fatal out-

come; in those who survive, neurological sequelae such as motor disability or mental retardation are common. In the compromised host a
widely disseminated disease can occur which may
be fatal.

C. DIAGNOSIS.
    1. _Clinical_. A diagnosis of cytomegalo-
virus infection should be considered in all infants with jaundice or signs similar to those
previously given. The exact diagnosis can only
be established in association with laboratory
data.
    2. _Laboratory_.
        a. Isolation of the Virus. The virus
may be isolated in cultures of human fibroblasts
such as WI-38 cells. Specimens from which it
may be cultured are urine, saliva, blood, nasopharyngeal and throat swabs antemortem, and the
involved organ postmortem. In mononucleosis it
may be isolated from peripheral leucocytes.
Characteristic focal cytopathology and inclusion
bodies develop in the infected cells after an
incubation period of 1 to 2 weeks. Identification is then carried out by serological methods.
Virus isolation is the method of choice to demonstrate a current active clinically apparent or
asymptomatic infection. Demonstration of a
viruria in the infant immediately after birth is
sufficient evidence for a diagnosis of a congenital infection.
        b. Serology. Complement fixation and
indirect FA tests may be used to help establish
a diagnosis. The CF test is most often used. In
the case of a primary infection a diagnosis may
be established on the basis of a fourfold or
greater increase in serum antibody titer during
convalescence. However, many infections seen
clinically are those that are either reinfections
or those that have been acquired prenatally and
therefore do not fit into this category. In the
case of reinfection a diagnosis still may be
established if the acute serum specimen is collected on the first or second day following the
appearance of clinical signs and symptoms. A

serum specimen collected 10 to 14 days later
would then show a significant increase in cytomegalovirus antibody over a pre-existing acute
serum base level. Maternal IgG cytomegalovirus
antibody may be present in the serum of neonates,
and it is necessary to prove the presence of IgM
antibody (produced by the fetus *in utero*) in the
newborn to establish a diagnosis of a prenatal
infection by serological methods. This requires
the use of an indirect or immunofluorescent test
which is not routinely done in most laboratories.
The total IgM level *per se* may be elevated but
this in itself is not diagnostic since it also
occurs in other prenatal infections. A more
specific test which is considered indicative of
a prenatal infection involves the demonstration
of a high level of specific cytomegalovirus IgM
antibody in the newborn's serum by the afore-
mentioned IFA test.

     c. Inclusion Bodies. The detection of
characteristic cytomegalovirus inclusion bodies
in cells collected from centrifuged urine or
gastric washings is pathognomonic of this disease.
Postmortem they may also be found in lung, liver,
and salivary gland tissue. The pathological
findings must be evaluated in association with
clinical signs and symptoms since it has been
shown in some studies that from 10 to 18 percent
of all infants autopsied (for reasons other than
cytomegalovirus infection) may have similar
lesions.

D. TREATMENT. There is no specific treatment
for this disease. Adenine arabinoside (Ara-A),
a purine nucleoside, has undergone a few tests
in humans to determine its effectiveness in the
treatment of cytomegalovirus infections which
were congenital or which appeared after immunosuppression or as mononucleosis. The results
indicated that Ara-A at subtoxic human levels
was virustatic and produced a reduction in virus
excretion. The response was least favorable in
immunosuppressed patients.

E.   EPIDEMIOLOGY.   Cytomegalovirus disease is
worldwide in distribution and has no particular
seasonal incidence.   There are two well-known
methods of transmission: 1) Transplacental, due
to a primary or reactivated infection in the
mother, and 2) transfusion of large volumes of
fresh whole blood.   In addition, it is probable
that the vast majority of the subclinical infections are acquired by direct contact with
saliva or respiratory secretions from subclinical cases.   Transnatal (during passage down the
birth canal) infection also now appears to be a
means by which infection takes place.   It has
been shown that a maternal viruria was present
at the time of delivery in 3 to 4 percent of those
tested.   It was also determined that approximately
10 to 13 percent of a series of babies examined
proved to have a viruria in the period of 3 to
12 months of age.   In the general population, by
age 2 years 14 percent of the persons tested had
demonstrable antibody; by age 25, 53 percent; and
by age 35, 81 percent.   Yet, overt clinical disease due to this virus is uncommon.

F.   PREVENTION.   Neither active nor passive immunization is practiced for the prevention of this
disease.

G.   CONTROL.   There are no specific or general
control measures.

Chapter X

HERPES SIMPLEX VIRUS (HERPESVIRUS HOMINIS)

A. PROPERTIES OF THE VIRUS. Herpes simplex virus contains DNA as its genetic material, is approximately 110 nm in size, is enveloped, and has a typical herpes group cubic icosahedral symmetry. There are two closely related antigenic types which can be identified by neutralization, herpes simplex virus types 1 and 2 (HSV-1 and HSV-2). Herpes viruses are inactivated readily by ether, chloroform, phenol and formaldehyde but remain viable for years when frozen at -70°C.

B. HOST RESPONSE TO INFECTION.
 1. *Incubation Period, Signs and Symptoms*. The incubation period for both HSV-1 and HSV-2 is 2 to 20 days with an average of about 6 days. A relationship exists between the HSV type and the body tissue which is infected. The relationship is not absolute, but in general HSV-1 is responsible for infections of the eye, lips, oral cavity, central nervous system and skin above the waist. HSV-2 is most commonly associated with infections of the urogenital area and skin below the waist.
 a. Herpes Simplex Infection of the Skin and Mucous Membranes. Infections of the lips (herpes labialis) and mouth are the most common manifestations of HSV-1. The lesions are usually present as a group of closely related vesicles which last about a week. Scabs form and the eruption resolves without scar formation. In the mouth the lesions appear as small painful ulcerated areas. There is a tendency for these conditions to recur, and often the exacerbation is brought on by such factors as slight tissue trauma, sunlight or menstruation. Herpes gingivostomatitis is a severe and extensive infection of the gums, tongue, mouth, and pharynx. It is usually seen in children 1 to 3 years of age and the condition

is accompanied by a high fever and cervical
adenopathy.

     b. <u>Kaposi's Varicelliform Eruption or
Eczema Herpeticum</u>. This is a generalized pustular form of HSV infection which is most often
seen in children with a pre-existing eczema.
There are constitutional symptoms and a high
fever. This condition can be fatal if the virus
becomes disseminated to vital organs.

     c. <u>Meningoencephalitis and Encephalitis</u>.
This is usually a primary HSV infection that is
seen in children and young adults. The onset is
sudden with fever, chills, and headache. Patients
show signs of meningeal irritation and there are
alterations in reflexes and convulsions. The
disease may be fatal, with death occurring on
the 8th to 10th day after onset.

     d. <u>Keratoconjunctivitis</u>. This condition
may be caused by either a primary or recurrent
HSV infection. At the onset there is a sensation
of a foreign body in the eye, photophobia, tear-
ing, and pain. A clinical diagnosis of herpes
is suggested by typical dendritic corneal ulcers.
Healing may require several weeks. Occasionally
deeper layers of the cornea are involved (disci-
form keratitis) and there is an interstitial gray
corneal opacity. Herpes eye infections are probably the leading cause of corneal scarring in the
United States.

     e. <u>Genitourinary Herpes</u>. Genital infec-
tions are most often seen in young adults and are
due to venereally transmitted HSV-2. However,
autoinfection of the urogenital tract with HSV-1
may occasionally take place. About 5 to 10 percent of all genital herpes infections can be
shown to be due to HSV-1.*

----

*Recent evidence points to a possible shift in
  the incidence of genital herpes due to HSV-1 as
  compared with HSV-2. In a study of 21 genital
  HSV isolates that were typed, 11 were type 1
  and 10 were type 2. It has been suggested that
  orogenital sex may play a role in the increased
  incidence of HSV-1 genital infections.

In females the primary lesions may be few in number, heal, and not recur and no visit to a clinician is made. In other cases the vesicular lesions may be more extensive, and confluent ulcers form which cover the entire area surrounding the vulvar orifice. The lesions may recur and present a continuing problem. In males the vesicles are usually few in number and appear on the penis and prepuce.

      f. <u>Transnatal Herpes</u>. A complication of genital herpes is the infection of the fetus during passage down the birth canal. This often results in a fatal generalized herpes infection in the neonate. Evidence of herpes genital lesions up to 3 weeks prior to delivery is considered sufficient to warrant cesarean section. In a recent study it was shown that this procedure prevented neonatal herpes infection in 15 out of 16 cases.

      g. <u>Cancer of the Cervix</u>. Considerable interest has recently been generated in regard to the possible role of HSV-2 in cancer of the cervix. This malignancy has an increased incidence in lower socioeconomic groups, prostitutes, women who marry early or begin sexual activity early and have multiple partners or marriages. This epidemiologic pattern points to the possibility of a venereally transmitted etiologic agent. HSV-2 is such an agent and in addition has an interesting latency potential. Studies have shown that women with cancer of the cervix have a higher incidence of antibodies to HSV-2 than those without this condition. It has also been reported that there is an increased incidence of cervical anaplasia in women with a history of cervical herpes infection. Other research designed to determine whether or not there is more than a casual association between HSV-2 and cancer of the cervix is in progress.

    2. *Pathogenesis*. Herpes simplex infections most often take place by contamination of breaks in the skin or mucous membranes with the virus. There is a multiplication in the local tissue

and extension to the regional lymph nodes. A
viremia is uncommon except in the compromised
host or in the newborn. In these cases the
virus may be spread through the blood to all
organs. Following infection the virus may
remain localized in the neural tissue (sensory
ganglia) at the site of primary occurrence and
recur. The exact mechanism by which these
exacerbations take place is not known, but they
take place in the presence of serum antibody,
and are often brought on by such factors as
trauma, surgery, sunlight, drugs, etc. In
encephalitis the virus may undergo a neurogenic
or hematogenous spread to the brain where it
multiplies, especially in the cortex. Eye
infections result from direct implantation of
the virus on the cornea. Genital lesions may
be caused by autoinoculation of HSV-1 from
another body site, but most often are the result
of HSV-2 being directly implanted on the cervix
or penis during intercourse. The virus, once
again, normally remains localized at the primary
inoculation site.

    3. _Pathology_. The skin and mucous membrane
lesions of herpes show a ballooning degeneration,
cellular proliferation and acidophilic intranuclear inclusion bodies which are characteristic
of other herpes infections (varicella-zoster).
In encephalitis there is perivascular cuffing
and nerve cell destruction. In disseminated
herpes in the compromised host or newborn, all
organs may show focal necrosis and the presence
of intranuclear inclusion bodies.

    4. _Immune Response_. Neutralizing and com-
plement fixing antibodies, in primary infections,
may be detected at about 5 to 7 days, peak at
2 to 3 weeks and persist in low titer probably
for life. There is also a delayed hypersensitivity skin test reaction which may be elicited
with HSV antigen.

    5. _Prognosis_. Most persons are acquainted
with the irritating persistent HSV skin and lip
lesions. The outcome of these, as well as

infection of the mucous membranes, is always
favorable. Genital herpes, aside from its occasional implication as the cause of urethritis,
cystitis and prostatitis, is self-resolving in
the male, and when it occurs in the female, may
recur, but remains localized in the cervix.
Transnatally acquired herpes has a high mortality, and survivors usually show some neurological
sequelae. The same is true of herpes meningitis
or encephalitis where the disease may result in
death or permanent psychic or psychomotor disturbances. Eczema herpeticum can be severe and
presents special problems in regard to dehydration and secondary bacterial skin infection
which, without proper treatment, can be fatal.
Herpes keratoconjunctivitis is a severe and painful disease which may result in corneal scarring.

C.   DIAGNOSIS.
     1.   _Clinical_. The wide spectrum of clinical
manifestations of HSV makes clinical diagnosis
difficult and in certain cases (encephalitis,
meningitis, eczema herpeticum, conjunctivitis)
impossible. Characteristic lesions and their
tendency to recur or be brought on by a specific
tissue insult help to support an HSV diagnosis.
Herpes keratoconjunctivitis is suggested in all
cases of dendritic ulcers of the cornea. Transnatal herpes is to be suspected when the mother
has a history of genital herpes close to the time
of delivery.
     2.   _Laboratory_.
          a.   Isolation of the Virus. HSV may be
isolated in a wide variety of cells cultured
in vitro. These include human amnion, lung,
kidney, HeLa, KB and HEp #2 as well as rabbit
kidney. The virus produces characteristic "rounding up" of the cells at the periphery of the viral
plaques, and upon staining the cells show eosinophilic intranuclear inclusions. The virus may be
isolated from vesicle fluid, lesion scrapings
and the oropharynx. In cases of encephalitis and
meningitis the virus is only infrequently isolated
from cerebrospinal fluid. Specimens should be

collected within the first 5 days of infection,
and care must be taken to either inoculate cultures within hours of collection or refrigerate
or freeze the material. If the specimen is to
be shipped by mail, special transport medium is
required. The CPE and inclusion bodies of HSV
allow a presumptive identification to be made
usually within 48 hours after cell culture
inoculation. A specific identification of the
virus is based on neutralization, complement
fixation or immunofluorescence with specific
antiserum. Differentiation between HSV type 1
and 2 is not done by most clinical laboratories,
but when done it is best accomplished by means
of indirect hemagglutination inhibition, comparative neutralization, or immunofluorescence.
         b. Fluorescent Antibody. Direct or
indirect fluorescent antibody tests using HSV
antiserum may be performed on either lesion or
tissue culture material.
         c. Serology. Two commonly used serologi-
cal tests are neutralization and complement fixation. Both of these antibodies appear by the
end of the first week of the disease and peak at
2 to 3 weeks. Serum should be collected as early
as possible after infection and 10 to 14 days
later. Neutralization is more specific than
complement fixation, but in either case a standard fourfold increase in antibody titer is
diagnostic. Neither test is useful for diagnosis
when the disease recurs at short (months) intervals.

D. TREATMENT. For the most part treatment has
been supportive, such as daubing the lesions with
antiseptic solutions or preventing secondary
bacterial contamination by using antibiotics.
Others support the use of ether-saturated cotton
pressed on skin lesions several times a day.
Another method of treatment that is occasionally
used is the application of proflavine or neutral
red to the lesions followed by exposure to light
(photoinactivation).

E. CHEMOTHERAPY. The drug 5-iodo-2-deoxy-
uridine (IDU) has been used with variable suc-
cess in the treatment of herpes keratitis. It
is instilled in the eye as a 0.1 percent solution at 2-hour intervals for several days. In
cases of transnatal herpes or severe herpes
encephalitis IDU has been given systemically,
sometimes with dramatic results. Other drugs
which are under test are 1-B-D-arabinosylcyto-
sine (Ara-C) and 9-B-arabinosyladenine (Ara-A).

F. EPIDEMIOLOGY.
    1. _Herpes Simplex Type 1_. Primary infec-
tion takes place mainly between the ages of 1 and
3 years, and by 5 years of age 70 to 90 percent
possess antibodies to this virus. The incidence
is higher at an earlier age in lower socioeconomic groups, presumably owing to poorer hygiene
and crowded living conditions. The virus may be
excreted in the saliva for up to 7 weeks following
a primary infection. Transmission is by direct
contact with either subclinical, primary or
recurrent infections, and most often takes place
by way of the oro-respiratory route. It is also
possible that there is a low degree of transmission by fomites. Approximately 80 to 90 percent of the primary infections are subclinical,
and epidemics rarely occur. Man is the only
known reservoir, and the disease has no seasonal
incidence. In the case of recurrent infections
the exacerbation is the result of expression of
latent herpes virus brought on by certain conditions (sunlight, trauma, etc.).
    2. _Herpes Simplex Type 2_. HSV-2 is spread
venereally and primary infection occurs during
the age of maximal sexual activity. The incidence,
as with HSV-1, is higher in lower socioeconomic
groups. Antibodies to HSV-2 are rarely present
in females under age 10 to 14 years, but rapidly
reach a level of 40 to 70 percent by age 20 to
30 years. Similar information in regard to
males is not available, but would be expected to
follow a similar pattern.

G.   PREVENTION.

   1.   *Artificial Passive Immunization*. Passive
protection is not practiced with either HSV-1 or
HSV-2.

   2.   *Artificial Active Immunization*. Active
immunization is not routinely practiced. Three
HSV-1 and one HSV-2 inactivated virus vaccines
have been tested in humans. One is produced in
France (HSV-1), one in Germany (HSV-1 and HSV-2)
and one in America (HSV-1). Reports by some
investigators indicate that the HSV-1 vaccines
may be helpful in preventing HSV-1 but not HSV-2
recurrence. Information on the effectiveness of
the HSV-2 vaccine in preventing HSV-2 recurrences
is not available.

H.   CONTROL. There are no specific control
methods. Persons with eczema should be kept away
from known herpes cases.

Chapter XI

INFECTIOUS MONONUCLEOSIS

A. PROPERTIES OF THE INFECTIOUS AGENT. The
etiology of infectious mononucleosis or "glandular fever" has not been conclusively established. However, there is substantial clinical
and epidemiologic evidence implicating the
Epstein-Barr virus (EBV) as the causative agent
of this lymphoproliferative disease. EBV is a
member of the DNA-containing herpesvirus group.
On electron microscopic examination, EBV is
morphologically indistinguishable from other
members of the herpesvirus group (HSV, CMV,
V-Z), the virion consisting of a central nucleic
acid core with cubic capsid symmetry, and an
outer envelope. EBV has a predilection for
lymphoblastoid cells and is capable of trans-
forming peripheral lymphoid cells into "EBV-
carrier" cell lines which can be continuously
cultivated. Normal lymphoid cells do not survive extended cultivation. Attempts to cultivate EBV in epithelial or fibroblast cells have
been unsuccessful.

B. HOST RESPONSE TO INFECTION.
    1. *Clinical Picture*.
        a. Incubation Period. On the basis of
epidemiologic contact data, the incubation period
for infectious mononucleosis is probably 30 to
50 days in adults, and considerably shorter in
children (probably 10 days).
        b. Signs and Symptoms. Prodromal signs
and symptoms include headache, malaise, and
fatigue. Prominent clinical findings during the
acute phase of illness are: sore throat, cervical lymphadenopathy, and fever. In adults,
an erratic febrile course of one week or longer
may occur with temperatures peaking to 102° to
103°F in the late afternoon or evening. The
febrile period is shorter or may be absent in

children. Additional clinical features found in
lesser frequency are: palatine petechiae at
the soft and hard palate junction, splenomegaly,
hepatomegaly, and possible jaundice. In children,
and less so in adults, a rubelliform, or possibly
a scarlatiniform, hemorrhagic, or an urticarial
rash may appear early in the course of illness.

      c. _Prognosis_. Infectious mononucleosis
occurs mainly in adolescents and young adults.
The majority of the patients recover after about
2 to 3 weeks of illness without any major complications. The clinical illness may be more
severe and prolonged in individuals over 40 years
of age. Complications such as splenic rupture,
toxemia, pneumonia, and neurologic sequelae
(aseptic meningitis, encephalitis, Guillain-Barré
syndrome) have been infrequently reported.

    2. _Immune Response_.

      a. _Heterophil Antibody_. Unique heter-
ophil hemagglutinins of the IgM class usually
appear in infectious mononucleosis during the
first week of illness. The heterophil agglutinins for sheep and horse erythrocytes which
develop in infectious mononucleosis differ from
those found in normal sera (Forssman antibody)
and in cases of serum sickness. Differential
absorption of patient's serum with guinea pig
kidney tissue and bovine erythrocytes distin-
guishes the various heterophil agglutinins.

      1) Infectious mononucleosis--
hemagglutinin absorbed by bovine erythrocytes
and not by guinea pig kidney tissue.

      2) Normal (Forssman)--hemagglutinin
absorbed by guinea pig kidney tissue and not by
bovine erythrocytes.

      3) Serum sickness--hemagglutinin
not removed by either absorbent.

    The heterophil agglutinins in infectious
mononucleosis attain peak levels in about 4
weeks and persist for up to 6 months, occasionally for longer periods. In some clinically consistent cases of infectious mononucleosis in
young adults, and particularly children, the
heterophil antibody response may be transient or
undetectable.

   b. EBV Antibody. Specific EBV antibody
which is serologically distinct from heterophil
antibody develops in patients with infectious
mononucleosis. The EBV antibody appears early
during the acute phase of illness and is of the
IgM class. Following primary infection, a persistent carrier state is established in the
lymphoreticular system. EBV-IgG antibody demonstrable by IFA, CF and Nt methods appears
against the viral capsid antigen and persists for
many years. EBV is present in the oropharynx for
several weeks to many months after appearance of
serum antibody and probably persists for years
in the latent state. Other EBV-associated lymphoproliferative disorders in which specific
EBV antibody has been regularly found are
Burkitt's lymphoma and nasopharyngeal carcinoma.
A large segment of the normal adult population
with no apparent history of infectious mononucleosis has EBV antibody, signifying the high prevalence of subclinical infections in childhood.
Seroepidemiologic investigations show a correla-
tion between immunity to infectious mononucleosis
and presence of EBV antibody.
   3. Pathology. Widespread lymphoreticular
cell proliferation occurs in the majority of
clinically manifest cases of infectious mononucleosis. Abnormal mononuclear cell infiltrates consisting of a variety of lymphoid cells are prom-
inently found in the tonsils, liver, spleen, and
affected lymph nodes. A marked mononuclear
infiltration is evident in the bone marrow.

C. DIAGNOSIS.
   1. Clinical. The typical picture is that of
a young adult complaining of fatigue and presenting with the clinical triad of membranous tonsillopharyngitis, cervical lymphadenopathy, and
fever. ` Clinical findings indicative of infectious
mononucleosis are confirmed by hematologic, liver
enzyme, and serologic studies.
   2. Laboratory.
   a. Hematologic. Leukocyte counts are
usually elevated during the second week of illness

(wbc = 10,000 to 30,000/mm^3). The differential
leukocyte count shows over 50 percent lympho-
cytosis with presence of abnormal or atypical
lymphocytes, the so-called Downey cells.
  b. <u>Biochemical</u>. Although hepatomegaly
may not be evident, the majority of patients
with acute illness show elevation of serum
transaminase (SGOT, SGPT) and LDH levels.
  c. <u>Serologic</u>.
   1) Heterophil antibody--the differential absorption test (Davidsohn) with
bovine erythrocytes and guinea pig kidney tissue is routinely employed. This test is a modification of the original sheep erythrocyte
heterophil agglutination test (Paul-Bunnell).
The heterophil antibody associated with infectious mononucleosis appears during the acute
stage of illness. In some individuals, the
heterophil antibody response may be delayed
and additional testing at about 3 to 4 weeks
following onset of illness increases the frequency of serologic detection. Consistently
heterophil-negative cases occur, and are encoun-
tered more commonly in pediatric patients.
   2) Epstein-Barr virus antibody--
EBV antibody determinations are helpful in
establishing specific virologic diagnosis,
particularly in heterophil antibody-negative
patients. A variety of serologic techniques
have been employed for assay of serum EBV antibody, including agar gel diffusion, complement-
fixation, indirect immunofluorescence, and
membrane fluorescence. The indirect fluorescent antibody (IFA) method is most widely used
and employs EBV-infected lymphoid cell lines
as a substrate for the test. EBV antibody
titers of over 1:80 are usually found after the
first week of illness. Demonstration of a significant fourfold rise (or appearance) in antibody titer is not always possible owing to the
early appearance of EBV antibody. Presence of
EBV-specific IgM antibody by IFA would establish primary infection in infectious mononucleosis.

d. <u>Viral Isolation</u>. Isolation of EBV
in cell culture is not routinely attempted.
Replication of EBV is apparently restricted to
cells of the lymphoid series. The virus has been
found in peripheral leukocytes of patients with
infectious mononucleosis.

D. TREATMENT. No specific therapy is available.
Therapy is symptomatic and consists mainly of
bed rest. Physical sports should be restricted
to prevent possible splenic rupture.

E. EPIDEMIOLOGY.
   1. _Transmission and Communicability_. A
persistent EBV-carrier state is established in
the lymphoid tissues of the oropharynx following
infection, indicating that the main source of
transmission is the pharyngeal secretions.
Transmission by blood transfusion is possible.
Infectious mononucleosis is not a highly contagious disease and requires close personal contact
for its transmission. Its communicability by
intimate oral contact between adults has led to
its designation as the "kissing disease."
Salivary exchange may play an important role in
transmission.
   2. _Epidemiologic Features_. Age, socioeconomic conditions, and geography are important
factors in the epidemiology of infectious mononucleosis. EBV seroepidemiologic surveys reveal
that inapparent or subclinical infections are
common in childhood. The frequency of childhood
infection is directly related to poor hygienic
conditions and close and continuous contact.
With better living standards, primary EBV infection is postponed or delayed until adolescence
and adulthood. It is in the 15 to 24 year age
group who have escaped primary childhood infection that the majority of clinically manifest
cases of infectious mononucleosis occur, especially among college students. No distinctive
seasonal patterns have been found except for a
higher morbidity on college campuses in the
early fall and spring when social encounters are

presumably greater. Infectious mononucleosis
occurs in most countries in the world. In certain circumscribed geographic areas, e.g.,
central Africa, EBV infection is closely associated with another lymphoproliferative disorder,
Burkitt's lymphoma, a tumor found mainly in male
children.

F. PREVENTION AND CONTROL. There are no specific methods recommended for prevention and control
of infectious mononucleosis.

Chapter XII

VARICELLA (CHICKENPOX), HERPES ZOSTER (SHINGLES)

A. PROPERTIES OF THE VIRUS. Varicella and zoster are two different disease syndromes caused by the same virus (varicella-zoster virus). It contains DNA as its genetic material, has a cubic icosahedral symmetry, is enveloped and approximately 110 nm in size. It is classified as a member of the herpesvirus group. It does not possess a hemagglutinin and there is only one known antigenic type. It is inactivated by ether, chloroform or 56°C for 30 minutes. Viability of the virus decreases rapidly even when stored at -70°C, and complete inactivation may occur by about 3 months.

B. HOST RESPONSE TO INFECTION.
    1. _Varicella (chickenpox)_.
        a. <u>Incubation Period, Signs and Symptoms</u>. The incubation period is about 14 to 16 days and there are usually headache, malaise and a low grade fever preceding the skin eruption. The rash first appears on the trunk and spreads rapidly to the limbs, face and scalp. The lesions are 1 to 3 mm in diameter and pass through the stages of being macular (red spot), papular (pimple) and finally vesicular (fluid-filled). After a few days the vesicles dry up, a scab forms and drops off and healing without scarring takes place. The rash occurs in successive crops so that there are lesions in various stages (macular, papular and vesicular) within a given skin area. By about a week after their first appearance all will have reached the scab-forming stage. Fever is present throughout the period of the skin eruption and tends to be more severe in proportion to the extent of the rash.
        b. <u>Pathogenesis</u>. The probable route of varicella infection is by way of the upper respiratory tract. The virus multiplies in

respiratory tissue and regional lymph nodes and
penetrates into the blood stream, a viremia ensues, and the virus localizes in ectodermal tissue and mucosa. It is possible that the virus
also reaches the sensory ganglia where it remains
in a latent form.

        c. Pathology. The vesicles in varicella
disease are due to a ballooning degeneration of
the prickle cells (stratum germinativum) of the
skin. These cells become large in size (giant
cells) and contain eosinophilic intranuclear
inclusion bodies. There is little tendency to-
wards reticular (net-like) formation. In fatal
cases in infants postmortem examination has shown
similar changes in cells of the liver, pancreas,
lungs and other internal organs.

        d. Immune Response. Infection with
varicella virus gives rise to the production of
neutralizing (Nt) and complement fixing (CF)
antibodies which may be first detected at about
7 to 10 days post-rash. They peak at about
14 days, remain level for a few weeks and slowly
decline. The CF antibodies drop much more
rapidly than the Nt antibodies, and are undetectable after about a year. The Nt antibodies
persist for years, perhaps for life. Second
attacks of chickenpox in a normal host are
unknown. It must be remembered, however, that
zoster is a different disease manifestation of
a primary varicella infection.

        e. Prognosis. Chickenpox is a mild,
rarely fatal disease and complete recovery is the
rule. Problems may arise when, owing to scratch-
ing, the lesions become superinfected. Chickenpox encephalitis is rare, and when it occurs is
mild and normally self-resolves without sequelae.
When infection takes place during or shortly
after birth the virus may be widely disseminated
in the internal organs, resulting in death. Congenital infections occur and have a high mortality (21 percent). Varicella pneumonia may also
be a complication, which, though uncommon, is seen
most often in adult females. Infection in preg-

nancy may have an increased morbidity and
mortality.

    2.   *Zoster*.

        a.   <u>Incubation Period, Signs and Symptoms</u>.
Present concepts hold that zoster arises from
activation of varicella-zoster virus which, following a primary chickenpox infection, has localized in a latent state in the spinal ganglia.
The period between the primary infection and the
disease "zoster" may be many years. Four to
five days prior to the appearance of the rash
there are fever, malaise, and pain and tenderness along the involved dorsal nerve routes. The
rash which follows is unilateral over 99 percent
of the time, and appears along the endings of the
intercostal sensory nerves. It is first seen on
the trunk near the sternum or spine and spreads
outward along the involved nerves. The vesicles
are somewhat larger but otherwise indistinguishable from those of chickenpox. The striking
feature of zoster is its unilateral nature, with
the rash stopping abruptly at midline. The trunk
and face are most often involved but lesions may
also be present on the scalp and tongue. The
duration of the disease is variable, but in most
cases the vesicles dry up and crust over within
2 to 3 weeks after onset.

        b.   <u>Pathogenesis</u>. The varicella-zoster
virus localizes in the spinal ganglia in a latent
state following a primary infection and remains
suppressed by a low level of circulating antibody.
Any interference with this natural cycle by traumatic tissue insult, drug-induced antibody depres-
sion (such as by corticosteroids) or certain
diseases (tuberculosis, cancer) might result in
viral replication in the ganglionic cells. The
characteristic rash would then result from passage of the virus along the nerve fibers to the
skin.

        c.   <u>Pathology</u>. The pathology of the
lesions seen in zoster is the same as that of
varicella.

d. Immune Response. In zoster the specific antibody produced is in the immunoglobulin
G (IgG) fraction of the serum. Since IgG is the
antibody which is produced as a result of a
second contact (secondary response) with an antigen, this would bear out the theory of the pathogenesis of the disease. Complement fixing antibodies may be detected as early as the fourth
day after onset, peak at about two weeks, and
decline to where they are not detectable at about
a year. Neutralizing antibodies follow the same
pattern but persist for a much longer period of
time. The incidence of zoster is quite low
(about 3 to 4/1000 persons annually) and second
and even third attacks have been known to occur.

e. Prognosis. Zoster is more severe in
adults than in children, but in both groups it
usually resolves spontaneously without sequelae.
The most common complaint is a persistent neu-
ralgia which occurs in about 10 percent of all
cases in patients over age 40. Other complications involve the eye (*Zoster opthalmicus*), which
may result in scleritis and keratitis and leuco-
encephalitis and occasional pneumopathies.
Zoster is particularly severe and sometimes fatal
when associated with malignant diseases such as
leukemia or Hodgkin's.

C. DIAGNOSIS.
1. *Varicella*.
a. Clinical Diagnosis. The differential
diagnosis of varicella is made on the basis of
the type, location, distribution and sequence of
the rash.
b. Laboratory.
1) Isolation of the virus--varicella-
zoster virus cannot be grown in laboratory animals
but can be isolated and grown in cell cultures
of human amnion or foreskin or embryonic kidney,
thyroid, lung, or other tissues. The best specimen is vesicle fluid collected aseptically, and
it should be inoculated immediately into cell

cultures. When this is not possible the virus
should be suspended in sterile skim milk or nutrient broth and frozen at -70ºC.

2)   Serology--complement fixation
titrations are done using acute serum collected
early after disease onset and 10 to 14 days
later. A fourfold or greater varicella-zoster
antibody increase is diagnostic in the absence
of a simultaneous rise in herpes simplex antibody. Neutralization titrations are rarely done
owing to difficulty in keeping viable virus and
the time consuming nature of the test.

3)   Inclusion bodies--smears made of
material collected from the base of a vesicle
are treated with Giemsa stain and examined for
the presence of multinucleated giant cells containing eosinophilic intranuclear inclusions.

2. *Zoster*.

a.   Clinical Diagnosis. Diagnosis is
based on the typical varicella-zoster rash, the
unilateral nature of its distribution and the
pain which accompanies the eruption. It is also
helpful to remember that the disease does not
occur in epidemics and occurs with equal frequency
in males and females.

b.   Laboratory.
1)   Isolation of the virus--the
technique for virus isolation is the same as that
for varicella.

2)   Serology--serological techniques
are rarely used in the diagnosis of zoster. Complement fixing activity is detectable within a
few days of the appearance of the rash.

3)   Inclusion bodies--the method and
sought for results are the same as those given
for varicella.

D.   TREATMENT.
1. *Varicella*. Treatment is symptomatic.
If secondary bacterial contamination of the lesions
takes place, appropriate antibiotic therapy should
be instituted.

2. *Zoster*. There is no specific treatment
for zoster. The lesions should be kept free of
bacterial contamination, but if secondary infection occurs, it may be treated with the appropriate antibiotic. Chemotherapy with 5-iodo-2-
deoxyuridine has not been uniformly successful.

E.   EPIDEMIOLOGY.
1. *Varicella*. This disease is highly contagious and worldwide in distribution. The
largest number of cases occur in the winter and
spring in the 5 to 7 year age group. It is seen
with equal frequency in males and females, and
greater than 90 percent of adults are immune by
virtue of having had a natural infection. The
disease may be spread from shortly before until
7 days after the onset of the rash. It is
spread person to person by aerosols of oral
secretions of infected individuals. Man is the
only known reservoir. Transplacental infections
can occur.
2. *Zoster*. This disease is assumed to arise
from a latent infection and epidemics do not
occur. The incidence is about 3 cases per 1000
population per year and it is seen with equal
frequency in males and females. Although zoster
may occur in children, the largest number of cases
are seen after the age of 20 years with the peak
incidence in the 50 to 80 age group. There is
no particular seasonal relationship. In spite of
the fact that zoster can initiate epidemics of
varicella in nonimmune children, this seldom
happens. This may be due to the rare occurrence
of the virus in the respiratory secretions in
zoster, and the difficulty of transmission which
would have to be by vesicle fluid.

F.   PREVENTION.
1. *Varicella*.
a.   Artificial Active Immunization. There
is no vaccine available for varicella.
b.   Passive Immunization. Passive protection is not routinely practiced to prevent

varicella.   However, there is a preparation called
zoster immune globulin (ZIG) available for special cases from the Center for Disease Control
(CDC), Atlanta, Georgia.   Zoster immune globulin
is obtained by collecting zoster convalescent
plasma for fractionation of IgG.   It is collected
from adults, otherwise in good health, from 14
to 35 days after the onset of the exanthem.
Patients eligible for ZIG prophylaxis are children
with predisposing high risk conditions (leukemia
or lymphoma, an immunodeficiency syndrome, or
treatment with immunosuppressive drugs) who
have been exposed to an active case of varicella
within the preceding 72 hours.   A list of regional ZIG consultants may be obtained from CDC.
    2.   _Zoster_.
        a.   Active Immunization. No vaccine is
available for zoster.
        b.   Passive Immunization. Passive pro-
phylaxis is not practiced.

G.   CONTROL.
    1.   _Varicella_.   There is no specific control
available.   Known cases should be kept away from
infants and persons with predisposing high risk
conditions..
    2.   _Zoster_.   Control recommendations are the
same as those for varicella.

Chapter XIII

WARTS (VERRUCA)

A. PROPERTIES OF THE VIRUS. The virus of warts contains DNA as its genetic material, has a cubic symmetry, is 40 to 55 nm in size and does not have an envelope. It is classified as a member of the papovavirus group. Since the virus has not been grown in the laboratory, data on its biologic properties are not known.

B. HOST RESPONSE TO INFECTION.
  1. _Incubation Period, Signs and Symptoms_.
The incubation period in the case of natural infections is not known. There are two clinical types of warts, verruca vulgaris and verruca plana. The former may occur on any body area but is most commonly seen on the fingers and hands as small (one to several millimeter) epidermal tumors which are rough, elevated, firm to palpation and often occur in groups. They may remain stable for years or disappear spontaneously. Verruca plantaris (plantar warts) is a clinical subvariety of verruca vulgaris which involves the weight-bearing points of the body and is usually found beneath a callus. Because of this, and the persistent pressure of walking, they grow in depth and cause acute pain. Condyloma acuminatum is another clinical form of verruca vulgaris which involves the warm moist areas of the body, particularly the external genitalia. In appearance the lesions are large, red, soft masses which may coalesce. Verruca plana (juvenile warts), like verruca vulgaris, is most common in children. The lesions are always multiple and occur on the face, neck, and dorsal surfaces of the hands and arms. Unlike vulgaris, they are flat and smooth, they may remain unchanged for months or years, or disappear spontaneously.

   2.   *Pathogenesis*. The virus enters the body
through the skin following direct contact with
warts *per se* or contaminated materials.   It
remains localized in the skin and a viremia has
never been demonstrated.
   3.   *Pathology*. Microscopic examination of
verruca vulgaris lesions shows hyperkeratosis
and areas of acanthosis, papillomatosis and
parakeratosis.   The granular layer is thickened
and there are large vacuolated cells in the
outer layers of the stratum spinosum and granular layer.   In verruca plana, papillomatosis
and parakeratosis are rare and epidermal cell
vacuolation is much greater.
   4.   *Immune Response*. Very little information
in regard to the immune response to verruca is
available.   It has been shown, however, that
complement fixing antibodies develop in approximately half of all cases.
   5.   *Prognosis*. Warts are small benign tumors
which usually remain localized in the area of
the primary infection.   They may remain stable
for months, years, or for life, or they may
spontaneously regress and disappear.   Plantar
warts present a special problem since they occur
on the soles of the feet, and surgical intervention may be necessary.

C.   DIAGNOSIS.
   1.   *Clinical*. Clinical diagnosis of verruca
vulgaris and plana is usually not made since the
lesions are so common and easily recognized by
the layman.   Verruca plantaris is more difficult
to diagnose since the lesions usually occur
beneath calluses.   All painful calluses should
be suspected of containing a wart.   Diagnosis of
warts is made on the basis of the nature of the
gross and histologic (biopsy) aspects and location
of the lesions.
   2.   *Laboratory*.
      a.   Isolation of the Virus. The virus of
warts has not yet been propagated in the laboratory.
Papovavirus particles can be visualized by electron microscopy in biopsies of lesions.

     b.   <u>Serology</u>. Serological tests are not used as aids for the diagnosis of verruca.

D.   TREATMENT. Treatment of warts is usually not necessary since they are benign and often spontaneously regress. In certain cases disappearance may be effected by suggestion alone. Other methods of treatment depend upon physical removal or destruction of the wart-infected tissue and include surgery, radiation, cryocauterization and electrodesiccation. In venereal warts application of podophyllin is quite successful.

E.   EPIDEMIOLOGY. Warts are spread person to person by direct contact with verruca-infected tissue or contaminated objects. Autoinoculation from one body site to another can take place. The disease is worldwide in distribution and man is the only reservoir. It is most commonly seen as a primary infection in children but can occur in older age groups. Contrary to popular opinion it is unrelated to handling toads.

F.   PREVENTION. There are no specific methods for the prevention of warts. Neither artificial active nor passive immunization is available.

G.   CONTROL. There are no specific methods for the control of wart infection.

Chapter XIV

MOLLUSCUM CONTAGIOSUM

A. PROPERTIES OF THE VIRUS. Molluscum contagiosum virus, a member of the poxvirus group, contains DNA as its genetic material and has a
complex capsid symmetry. It is brick shaped, approximately 230 by 300 nm in size, and possesses
an envelope. Despite the latter fact, it is not
sensitive to inactivation by ether or chloroform.
It has not been successfully propagated in the
laboratory.

B. HOST RESPONSE TO INFECTION.
    1. _Incubation Period, Signs and Symptoms_.
The incubation period of the natural infection
is 2 weeks to 2 months. The primary infection
consists of lesions which are small, multiple,
smooth, firm, umbilicated tumors. They are most
often seen on the face, forehead, eyelids or genital or anal area, but also may be found on the
back, arms, buttocks and inner thigh. Squeezing
of the lesion will express a granular core from
the umbilicated area. The tumors usually spontaneously regress in from 2 weeks to 2 years.
Recurrences are seen in a fair number of cases.
Generalized eruptions may occur as a complication of immunosuppresive therapy.
    2. _Pathogenesis_. The virus enters the body
through the skin and localizes in the basal layer
of the epithelium. A viremia has not been demonstrated.
    3. _Pathology_. Sections of tumors viewed
microscopically show a typical picture. As a
result of degeneration of the cells of the epi-
dermis as they advance through the other layers,
a cavity forms in the center of the growth.
Cytoplasmic inclusions may be found in cells of
the basal layers of the epithelium. These inclusions consist of virus particles and eventually
fill the entire cytoplasm.

4. *Immune Response*. The antibody response
is not well understood. It is known that complement fixing antibodies are produced, but
aside from this other investigations have been
hampered owing to the lack of a suitable laboratory substrate.
5. *Prognosis*. The lesions normally spontaneously regress within a period of weeks to
months. Recurrences occur.

C. DIAGNOSIS.
1. *Clinical*. Diagnosis is made on the basis
of the tumors being multiple, umbilicated and
easily enucleated.
2. *Laboratory*.
a. Isolation of the Virus. No suitable
animal or other substrate for virus isolation
exists.
b. Serology. Serological tests are of
little value as diagnostic aids.
3. *Inclusion Bodies*. The typical cytoplasmic inclusions (molluscum bodies) seen in cells
from the lesions are useful as an aid to diagnosis.

D. TREATMENT. Since the tumors usually regress
spontaneously it is advisable to delay treatment
and let nature take its course. If there is
some pressing reason for treatment, they may be
removed by curettage followed by cauterization
of the resulting wound with zinc chloride or
iodine.

E. EPIDEMIOLOGY. The disease is spread by
direct or indirect contact (fomites) with lesion
material. Epidemics within family groups have
been reported. It is worldwide in distribution
and oocurs more often in children than in adults.
Humans are the only known virus reservoir.

F. PREVENTION. There is no specific method of
prevention.

G. CONTROL. There is no specific control method.
Care should be taken to disinfect objects which
come into contact with viral lesions.

Chapter XV

SMALLPOX (VARIOLA MAJOR)

A. PROPERTIES OF THE VIRUS. Variola virus contains DNA as its genetic material, is approximately 210 x 260 nm in size, possesses an envelope, has a complex symmetry and is classified as a member of the poxvirus group. It produces a hemagglutinin for chicken red blood cells, which is not an integral part of the virion, but which may be extracted from infected cells. There is only one antigenic type. The virus is very stable to drying and retains its infectivity on contaminated clothing and bed sheets for months. It is relatively resistant to 1 percent phenol but is inactivated by alcohol in about 1 hour at room temperature. It remains infective for years when stored at -20° to $-70^{\circ}C$.

B. HOST RESPONSE TO INFECTION.
   1. _Incubation Period, Signs and Symptoms_.
      a. Variola Major. The incubation period is 12 to 14 days and the first signs and symptoms are headache, backache, fever, chills and vomiting. These prodromata last for about 2 to 3 days, at which time the eruption appears, first on the face, and then on the extremities, palms, soles, trunk and buccal mucosa. The lesions are discrete papules which become vesicular after a few days and pustular after an additional 2 to 5 days. The temperature falls with the first appearance of the rash and returns at the time it becomes pustular. The lesions, unlike varicella, are all in the same stage at the same time. After an additional 2 to 6 days the lesions dry up, crusts form, and with their subsequent "falling off" leave small pink scars.
      b. Hemorrhagic Smallpox. This is a fulminating, often fatal, form of smallpox seen in a small percentage of cases. It has a short course, and patients usually die within 3 to 6

days after onset. There is hemorrhage into the
skin lesions and from the mucous membranes. A
characteristic smallpox vesicular eruption does
not develop.

      c. <u>Alastrim or Variola Minor</u>. This form
of smallpox is due to a virus strain of low virulence. The incubation period is slightly longer
than with variola major, but the disease is much
milder, seldom fatal, and the rash does not
become pustular.

      d. <u>Varioloid or Modified Smallpox</u>. An
abortive type of smallpox can occur in a previously immunized individual when the antibody
titer is low. The signs and symptoms are much
milder in nature and the rash is sparse and resembles that of chickenpox. The lesions may
become pustular but the systemic reaction is
absent.

      2. *Pathogenesis*. The virus enters by way
of the upper respiratory tract and multiplies in
the mucosa and lymphoid tissue. A transient low-
grade viremia results which serves to spread the
virus to the reticuloendothelial system (spleen,
liver, bone marrow). Viral replication in these
organs results in a second more extensive viremia
and infection of the epidermal cells of the skin
and mucous membranes.

      3. *Pathology*. The lesions *per se* in small-
pox are due to a focal degeneration of stratified
epithelium accompanied by a serous exudation and
vesicle formation. Stained specimens, collected
by scraping during the maculopapular stage, or
fluid collection during the vesicular stage show
the presence of spherical intracytoplasmic
inclusions. These inclusions, which are called
Guarnieri bodies, are acidophilic, usually 1 to
4 μ in size, surrounded by a halo and located
near the nucleus. They consist of virus particles and viral antigen. Guarnieri bodies may be
detected in lesion material for a period up to
6 days after the first appearance of the rash,
but are difficult to demonstrate in specimens
taken during the pustular stage. In man they are
found exclusively in lesions of the skin and

mucous membranes.

   4. *Immune Response*. Complement fixing antibodies may be detected at 8 to 10 days after onset of symptoms, peak at 2 to 3 weeks and disappear by 6 to 8 months. Hemagglutination inhibiting antibodies appear at 3 to 5 days, peak at
2 to 3 weeks and persist for years. Neutralizing
antibodies are present at about the 6th day after
onset, peak at 2 to 3 weeks and persist for years.
In patients with *modified smallpox* (those previously vaccinated) all 3 antibodies appear
earlier and reach higher titers than in those
who have never been vaccinated.

   5. *Prognosis*. The mortality varies from 1
to 40 percent depending upon the form of the
disease and the age of the patient. Less than
1 percent of variola minor infections are fatal,
compared with up to 40 percent of hemorrhagic
variola major infections. The disease is much
more severe in infants than in adults. Complications, which may be treated with antibiotics,
are contamination of the skin lesions or bronchopneumonia caused by bacteria. Encephalitis due
to the virus *per se* is rare. When infection
takes place during pregnancy the virus can reach
the fetus transplacentally, resulting in an
increased incidence of spontaneous abortions.
Scarring, which occurs when the crusts fall off,
can be extensive and present a cosmetic problem.

C. DIAGNOSIS.

   1. *Clinical*. The morphology, distribution
and sequence of development of the rash as described in "signs and symptoms" usually is sufficient to establish a differential diagnosis.
This determination is strengthened by an evaluation of the patient's history in regard to
previous vaccination or travel to or from an
endemic area. The modified form of smallpox
is often confused with varicella, but rigid
attention to the above serves to separate the
two. Laboratory assistance in verifying the
diagnosis is imperative.

2. *Laboratory*.
    a. <u>Isolation of the Virus</u>. Virus is present in the skin lesions from the time of first appearance through and including the period of scab formation. It is present in saliva only when there are well developed oral lesions on the mucous membranes. Isolation from the blood is not easy, even though it can be shown that the virus is present from the onset of rash through the period of pustule formation. The substrate of choice is the chorioallantoic membrane of 10 to 14 day old chick embryos. The virus produces pocks on this tissue and can be differentiated from vaccinia and herpes simplex viruses on the basis of pock morphology. Varicella-zoster virus does not grow on the chick embryo chorioallantoic membrane. The pock material may also be stained and examined for Guarnieri bodies, which are characteristic of variola-vaccinia. A minimum of 3 days is required to complete the above sequence. Smallpox virus may also be grown in human foreskin, HeLa, or monkey kidney cultures and produces hyperplastic foci which develop into small plaques following cell necrosis. The hyperplastic foci are not produced by vaccinia virus. Further differentiation of smallpox and vaccinia viruses is accomplished by the ability of the former to grow at 39° to $40^\circ C$, whereas vaccinia virus will grow only at a temperature several degrees lower. Varicella-zoster virus (herpesvirus group) is easily distinguished from the poxviruses in stained preparations.
    c. <u>Other Detection Aids</u>. Material from skin lesions can be tested directly for poxvirus particles by electron microscopic examination or by precipitation in agar gel. The agar gel precipitation test utilizes a known antivaccinial rabbit serum for detection of variola-vaccinia antigen.
    d. <u>Serology</u>. Serologic tests are of limited value because of the need for rapid diagnosis. Smallpox complement fixing, hemagglutination inhibiting, and neutralizing tests

may be used but antibodies do not appear until
about 7 days after onset of illness. A fourfold or greater increase in antibody titer would
be diagnostic.

D. TREATMENT. There is no specific treatment
for smallpox once the disease has developed.
Antibiotics may be used to prevent secondary
bacterial infection.

E. EPIDEMIOLOGY. Prior to the use of smallpox
vaccination the disease had a worldwide distribution and occurred in devastating epidemics.
It has been estimated that in the 18th century
in Europe two out of every ten children born
died of smallpox. Immunization has eradicated
the disease from most countries and it is now
endemic in Bangladesh, Botswana, Ethiopia, India,
Nepal, Pakistan and Sudan. The dramatic impact
of worldwide vaccination is further indicated by
its reduction of a total estimated 2.5 million
cases of smallpox in 1967 to 500,000 cases in
1971.
      When epidemics occur, persons of both sexes
and in all age groups, who are not immune by
virtue of vaccination or previous contact, may
be infected. The disease may be spread from the
onset of viremia (about 10 days after contact)
up to and including the time of formation of
crusts. Crusts which have fallen off may remain
infective for months. The disease is spread by
direct contact (respiratory secretions, skin
lesion contact), by fomites (bedding, clothes) and
in rare instances by transplacental passage. Man
is the only known reservoir of smallpox virus.

F. PREVENTION.
      1. *Active Immunization*.
            a. Vaccinia Virus. Artificial immuniza-
tion in man is accomplished by the use of live
vaccinia virus. The origin of the present vaccine virus is not known but three possibilities
exist: 1) vaccinia may be a separate virus
species; 2) it may represent a variola virus

which became attenuated by natural passage
through cows; 3) it may be a cowpox virus
which has been altered by laboratory passage.
At any rate, vaccinia virus is antigenically
very similar to variola virus and produces in
man a mild disease which produces a highly effective immunity against smallpox. The vaccine
is produced by the inoculation of vaccinia virus
on scarification sites on calves or sheep and
collecting the resulting lesion material following virus growth. It may also be produced in
chick embryos. The packaged product should have
no less than 10^8 live virus particles per ml.,
and is prepared in either a liquid, glycerinized
(40 percent glycerol) or lyophilized (dried)
form. Rigid attention must be paid to the manufacturer's instructions for storage and handling.

　　　　b.　Effectiveness. Successful vaccination confers a high level of protection for at
least 3 years, and a substantial but waning
immunity for 10 years or more.

　　　　c.　Vaccine Usage.

　　　　1)　General recommendations--the
routine use of smallpox vaccination for the
general public and as part of pediatric immunization schedules is no longer recommended in the
United States. This decision was made in 1971.
The risk of smallpox in the United States is
now considered to be so small that it is out-
weighed by the risk of complications which may
arise as a result of vaccination.

　　　　2)　International travelers--all
travelers going to endemic or infected areas
should be vaccinated. An endemic area is
defined as one where there is transmission of
uncontrolled nonimported smallpox in a population. An infected area is one where there
is transmission of secondary cases following an
importation.

　　　　3)　High risk groups--hospital and
health personnel should be vaccinated (and revaccinated every 3 years).

d.   Complications. An indication of the
risk involved in smallpox vaccination may be
seen in the statistics for the year 1968 in the
United States.   Among more than 5.6 million
primary vaccinees and 8.6 million revaccinees
and their contacts there were 16 cases of encephalitis, 11 cases of vaccinia necrosum and 126
cases of eczema vaccinatum. Nine persons died.
A substantial number of less serious complications
occurred.   It must be pointed out that the number
of complications could have been reduced by as
much as 50 percent if known contraindications
were heeded.   Complications were twice as high
in infants under 1 year of age as in all other
age groups.

e.   Contraindications. Any skin disorder
in the individual to be vaccinated or in household contacts is a contraindication to vaccine
use.   Pregnancy, altered immune states, leukemia,
lymphoma, therapy with immunosuppressive drugs
and radiation are also contraindications to use.
There is no evidence that smallpox vaccination
has any therapeutic value in the treatment of
recurrent herpes or warts.

f.   Vaccination Techniques.
1)   Site of vaccination--normally the
skin over the insertion of the deltoid muscle or
posterior aspect of the arm over the triceps
muscle is the preferred vaccination site.   The
skin may be cleansed with water and should be
dry prior to vaccination.

2)   Methods.
a)   Jet injection--the recom-
mended dose of vaccine is injected intradermally
by means of a jet injection apparatus.

b)   Multiple pressure--a small
drop of vaccine is placed on dry cleansed skin
and a series of 10 pressures for primary and
30 pressures for revaccination are made through
the vaccine with the side of a sterile needle.
No dressing should be applied.

c)   Multiple puncture--this
technique uses a sterile bifurcated needle

which is inserted into the vaccine to collect a
drop of fluid which is deposited on the cleansed
skin. A series of skin punctures are made
through the vaccine. (Using the bifurcated
needle technique a single vaccinator can perform
as many as 1500 vaccinations per day.)

     g. Interpretation of Responses.

     1) Time of inspection--it is now
recommended that the vaccination site be inspected
at 6 to 8 days after vaccination.

     2) Primary vaccination--a successful
primary vaccination is indicated by the presence
of a typical Jennerian vesicle.

     3) Revaccination--two types of re-
vaccination response are defined by the WHO Expert Committee on Smallpox, eliminating use of
older terms such as "accelerated" and "immune."
They are:

     Major reaction--a vesicular or
pustular lesion or an area of definite palpable
induration or congestion surrounding a central
lesion which may be a crust or an ulcer. This
reaction indicates that virus multiplication has
taken place and that the revaccination is successful.

     Equivocal reaction--all reactions
other than "major reactions." They may be the
consequences of immunity adequate to suppress
virus multiplication or may represent only allergic reactions to an inactive vaccine. If an
equivocal reaction is observed, revaccination procedures should be checked and vaccination repeated
with vaccine from another lot.*

     2. *Passive Immunization*. Passive protection
is not routinely practiced as a prophylactic
measure against smallpox. (See VIG, below.)

     3. *Vaccinia Immune Globulin (VIG)*. Gamma
globulin is collected by fractionating blood serum
of recently vaccinated individuals. It is pro-
vided by the Center for Disease Control and

---

* Supplement, Collected Recommendations of the
  Public Health Service Advisory Committee on
  Immunization Practices, 1972.

stored at nine Public Health Service Stations in the United States. It is available at no cost for treatment of the following conditions: eczema vaccinatum, progressive vaccinia, or autoinoculation vaccinia of the eye. It may also be helpful for severe cases of generalized vaccinia. It is not useful for post-vaccinial encephalitis. It is effective in conferring protection against smallpox if given shortly after exposure to the disease, but because it is in short supply and confers only temporary protection it is not a successful alternative to vaccination.

    4. _Chemotherapy_. Certain of the thiosemi-carbazone derivatives (N-methyl-isatin-B-thio-semicarbazone, Marboran) have been shown to be effective in the prevention of smallpox in contacts of cases. The protection is temporary and the drug has no effect when given once the disease is evident. Other chemotherapeutic agents are under study.

G. CONTROL. Vaccination is obviously the best method of controlling smallpox. In epidemics, diagnosed and suspected cases are kept in isolation. It is also important to locate contacts of known cases so that adequate preventive measures may be taken. All material which comes into contact with a smallpox case is sterilized. A certificate of recent vaccination or revaccination is required of all travelers to or from an endemic or infected area.

Part Three

RNA VIRUSES

Chapter XVI

LYMPHOCYTIC CHORIOMENINGITIS

A. PROPERTIES OF THE VIRUS. The virus has single stranded RNA as its genetic material, is about 50 nm in size, is enveloped and has a spherical or pleomorphic morphology. Its capsid symmetry has not been established. It is classified in a group called the Arenaviruses ("sandy") together with Lassa and the Tacaribe viruses. The virus is inactivated rapidly at 37°C, and slowly at refrigerator temperature. It may be preserved for several days at 0°C and for longer periods at -70°C. It is inactivated by lipid solvents or 0.1 percent formaldehyde, but is resistant to phenol.

B. HOST RESPONSE TO INFECTION.
   1. *Incubation Period, Signs and Symptoms*. The incubation period is 1 to 3 weeks. The infection in man may present as a mild influenza-like disease, aseptic meningitis or meningoencephalomyelitis. The most common type is either respiratory or meningeal. The disease is ushered in with fever, headache, and chills which may represent the total disease picture. In other cases there is a short period of remission followed by a recurrence of the original syndrome together with nausea, vomiting and signs of meningeal irritation. Recovery usually takes place within two weeks, and there are no sequelae. In those rare instances where the disease takes the form of a meningoencephalomyelitis there may be paralysis of the limbs, and sensory disturbances. Even in this case, however, complete recovery is the rule.
   2. *Pathogenesis*. The virus enters by way of the respiratory tract. A viremia is present during the acute stage and the virus is present in the kidney, spleen, liver and lung; in meningitis, in the meninges, ependyma, and choroid

plexus. The route by which the virus reaches
these tissues is not well known.

    3. *Pathology*. In fatal cases there are
inflammatory changes in the meninges, ventric-
ular ependyma and choroid plexuses due to infiltration with lymphocytes and macrophages. In
rare cases the brain may show perivascular cuffing, gliosis and degeneration of nerve cells.

    4. *Immune Response*. Complement fixing
antibodies appear 2 to 3 weeks after disease
onset, peak at 6 to 7 weeks in very low titer,
and begin a gradual decline. Neutralizing antibodies are present at significant levels at
about 7 weeks and persist for up to 5 years.

    5. *Prognosis*. Lymphocytic-choriomeningitis
is usually a mild influenza-like disease which
is self-resolving with no secondary complications.
When the disease takes the form of a meningitis
it is more severe, but again is self-resolving.
Temporary memory loss, headache, and persistent
stiff neck occur only occasionally. In those
rare cases where the disease appears as an acute
systemic form, with coma, or encephalomyelitis,
the mortality is high.

C. DIAGNOSIS.

    1. *Clinical*. A history which reveals a
febrile period followed by a remission prior to
signs and symptoms of meningeal irritation, as
well as knowledge of a possible exposure to mice
or hamsters, is helpful in diagnosis. The spinal
fluid cell count may range between 100 and 600
cells per cu mm, mostly lymphocytes. The spinal
fluid sugar is normal and the protein slightly
elevated. A clinical diagnosis should be substantiated by the laboratory.

    2. *Laboratory*.

        a. Isolation of the Virus. The virus
may be isolated from the blood from the onset of
symptoms for a period of about 2 weeks. It is
isolated with difficulty from the spinal fluid
and persists in low titer in the urine for some
time after it is no longer found in the blood.

Isolation may be accomplished by the use of tissue cultures of primary African green or rhesus monkey kidney cells or passaged human KB or HEp#2 cells. It may also be grown in white mice by intracerebral inoculation. Identification is carried out by neutralization with specific LCM antiserum.

       b. Serology. Complement fixation and neutralization tests may be carried out using acute (1st week) and convalescent serum. The CF antibodies appear at 2 to 3 weeks, but Nt antibodies do not become positive until 6 weeks after onset. In either case a fourfold increase in antibody titer is required for diagnosis. In meningitis cases antibody is detectable by indirect FA within one week after onset of CNS signs and symptoms.

D. TREATMENT. There is no specific treatment for LCM.

E. EPIDEMIOLOGY. The main reservoir is the house mouse, but the virus is also endemic in dogs, sheep, calves, monkeys, guinea pigs and hamsters. Lice and ticks may harbor the virus. Man is a chance host and is most likely infected by inhalation of contaminated mouse urine or feces. The portal of entry is the respiratory tract and there is no man to man transmission. The disease in humans occurs mainly in winter and spring, may occur as small outbreaks and is worldwide in distribution.

F. PREVENTION. There are no specific biological preventive measures. There is no vaccine in prospect and passive protection is not practical.

G. CONTROL. Control is strictly on the basis of eradication of the house mouse.

Chapter XVII

CORONAVIRUS

A. PROPERTIES OF THE VIRUS. These viruses contain RNA as their genetic material, are approximately 70 to 120 nm in size, spherical to pleomorphic with petal-shaped surface projections and possess an envelope. They are believed to have a helical symmetry and are the only members of the coronavirus group. Information on their physical and chemical properties is sparse, but it is known that they are quite labile and readily inactivated in solutions with a pH which varies by more than 0.5 on either side of 7.2. Three types have been identified on the basis of neutralization. Two strains have been shown to agglutinate red blood cells from man, mice, rats and chickens.

B. HOST RESPONSE TO INFECTION.
   1. *Incubation Period, Signs and Symptoms*.
The incubation period is about 3 days and the disease lasts for about a week. These viruses are responsible for acute respiratory diseases which cannot be distinguished clinically from the common cold.
   2. *Pathogenesis*. Very little is known about the pathogenesis of these viruses. They obviously enter by way of the upper respiratory tract and remain localized in that area. They have not been shown to involve the pulmonary tissues.
   3. *Pathology*. Since these viruses cause only mild nonfatal diseases the extent of their pathology is not known.
   4. *Immune Response*. The production of CF, Nt and HI antibodies follows infection, but how long they persist and whether or not they prevent homotypic reinfection is not known.
   5. *Prognosis*. The diseases caused by coronaviruses are mild and self-resolving and complete recovery within 6 to 7 days is the rule.

C.   DIAGNOSIS.
   1. _Clinical_. There are a wide variety of
viruses which can cause signs and symptoms similar to those produced by coronaviruses. Clinical diagnosis is not possible.
   2. _Laboratory_.
      a. Isolation of the Virus. Attempts to
isolate these viruses are usually not made because of the nature of the cell cultures needed
to perform an efficient job. Certain strains
grow only in organ cultures of ciliated human
embryonic nasal and tracheal tissues while others
may be isolated in human embryonic kidney cells.
      b. Serology. A fourfold increase in
coronavirus CF or HI antibody in serum specimens
collected early in the disease and convalescent
serum collected about 2 weeks after onset is
diagnostic.

D.   TREATMENT.   There is no specific treatment
for coronavirus infections.

E.   EPIDEMIOLOGY.   These viruses are spread
person to person by means of nasal secretions
from acute cases. Most infections occur in the
late winter or early spring. In contrast to parainfluenza virus infections, coronaviruses are
more commonly associated with upper respiratory
tract disease in adults. They are responsible
for about 10 to 20 percent of all adult common
cold-like syndromes.

F.   PREVENTION.   There are no specific methods
of prevention.

G.   CONTROL.   There are no specific control
measures which can be taken.

Chapter XVIII

INFLUENZA

A. PROPERTIES OF THE VIRUS.

 1. *Physico-Chemical Properties*. Influenza
virus possesses RNA as its genetic material,
measures 90 to 120 nm in size, and is a member
of the orthomyxovirus group. The viral RNA is
arranged in a helical pattern and contains spherical protein subunits. The helical ribonucleoprotein (nucleocapsid) is 9 nm in diameter and
is half the size of the ribonucleoprotein helix
of the paramyxoviruses. The nucleocapsid is
encased in a continuous membrane shell consisting of an internal protein layer (membrane protein) and an external lipid-containing envelope.
The hemagglutinating and enzymatic eluting
properties of the virus reside in distinct hemagglutinin and neuraminidase glycoprotein "spikes,"
approximately 9 nm in length, which are embedded
in and project from the surface of the envelope.
In the infectious process, the hemagglutinin
binds the virus to the cell, and following penetration and internal replication, the virus is
assembled and released from the cell membrane
by the action of the enzyme neuraminidase. An
RNA-dependent RNA polymerase (RNA transcriptase)
which plays a role in viral RNA synthesis has
been found associated with the virion. Influenza
virus is inactivated by ether, ultraviolet irradiation, acid and formaldehyde treatment. Heat-
ing at 56°C destroys viral infectivity but hemagglutinating activity remains intact. The virus
can be preserved in a viable state for years by
lyophilization or storage at -70°C.

 2. *Antigenic Properties*. Three antigenic
types of influenza virus, designated A, B and C,
have been found and include orthomyxoviruses of
human, swine, equine, and avian origin. The
type-specificity of influenza viruses is associated with a common ribonucleoprotein antigen

which is shared by all influenza virus strains
of a given type and which does not cross-react
between serotypes. Antigenic variation resulting in the development of new influenza virus
strains has been attributed to an "antigenic
shift" in the hemagglutinin and neuraminidase
components of the virus. The genetic alterations in the hemagglutinin and neuraminidase
antigens have occurred mainly with influenza A,
and less so with influenza B virus. Influenza
C virus has remained antigenically stable since
its initial isolation in 1947. Epidemics of
influenza A which have coincided with major antigenic shifts in the hemagglutinin and neuraminidase antigens are shown in Table 7. In inter-
epidemic years when influenza A occurs sporadically in focal outbreaks, minor antigenic
variants or intermediate strains are found, e.g.,
the recent "London flu" {Influenza A/England/
42/72 (H_3N_2)} and the Port Chalmers {Influenza
A/Port Chalmers/1/73 (H_3N_2)} viruses. The unique
genetic constitution of influenza A virus allows
for emergence of new or modified viral strains
by a process of genetic recombination presumably
as the population develops immunity to existing
strains. Although considerable antigenic variation has occurred with influenza B virus, the
antigenic demarcations are less distinctive than
with influenza A virus.

TABLE 7   Influenza A Viruses Associated with Major Epidemics

Major Subtypes*	Prevalence
A/Puerto Rico/8/34 (HON1)	1933-1946
A/Fort Monmouth/1/46 (H1N1)	1947-1957
A/Singapore/1/57 (H_2N_2)	1957-1967
A/Hong Kong/1/68 (H_3N_2)	1968-

*Antigenic / Geographic / Strain / Yr. of Iso- /
   type   /   origin   /   No. /   lation /

  (Antigenic character: Hemagglutinin, neuraminidase)

B.   HOST RESPONSE TO INFECTION.

   1.   *Signs* *and* *Symptoms*.   Influenza (la grippe)
is an acute respiratory disease with an abrupt
onset.   Following a short incubation period of
24 to 72 hours, there are sudden chills, fever,
headache, malaise, generalized myalgia, and, in
some cases, extreme exhaustion or prostration.
The conjuctivae and pharynx are injected and a
mild, nonproductive cough usually develops.   The
constitutional signs occur chiefly in influenza A
and are generally less pronounced in influenza B.
Influenza C infection usually manifests itself
as a mild upper respiratory illness.   The severity of influenza A and B varies according to an
individual's age and health status.   Mild upper
respiratory infection is common in healthy children and adults.   Infants and young children may
develop croup as a lower respiratory tract complication.   In the elderly, a serious influenzal
bronchopneumonia may develop which could be further complicated by bacterial superinfection.
Bacterial agents implicated in secondary pneumon-
ic infections are: *Staphylococcus aureus,*
Streptococcus pneumoniae (pneumococcus), beta-
hemolytic group A streptococci, and *Hemophilus*
influenzae.   Besides the elderly, persons of all
ages with chronic cardiovascular, pulmonary,
renal, and metabolic disorders are at high risk
of developing serious, and sometimes fatal,
illness.   Pregnant women may be at greater risk
of developing pulmonary complications.   Other
rare sequelae of influenza include encephalitis
and myocarditis or pericarditis.   Reyes' syndrome, an acute encephalopathy of as yet unknown
etiology, has occurred in children and adolescents as a rare complication of influenza B.

   2.   *Prognosis*.   In uncomplicated cases without lower respiratory tract involvement, the
fever lasts for 2 to 4 days and the patient
usually recovers in about one week after onset
of illness.   Easy fatigability may persist for
several weeks in older persons.   Serious prog-
nostic features are persistent fever, prolonged
prostration, and a complicating pneumonia.

Secondary bacterial pneumonias may be lethal and
must be promptly treated.

   3. *Immune Response*. Local secretory antibodies are believed to play a primary role in
preventing infection and spread of influenza
virus in the respiratory tract. Influenza virus
neutralizing and neuraminidase antibodies in the
respiratory secretions are associated with the
IgA class of immunoglobulins. Systemic or humoral antibodies of the IgM and IgG class become
detectable about one week after onset of illness
and attain peak levels at 2 to 4 weeks. Complement fixing antibodies appear against the
type-specific soluble ribonucleoprotein (S antigen) as well as the strain-specific viral component (V antigen). Hemagglutination inhibiting
(HI) and neuraminidase antibodies develop against
the hemagglutinin and viral enzyme glycoprotein
components, respectively. The humoral HI antibody persists at low levels for many years and
serves as an immunologic marker of an individual's
past influenza virus infection history. On reinfection with mutants of influenza A virus,
not only is HI antibody induced against the new
virus strain but an anamnestic antibody response
occurs against previously contacted antigenically
related strains ("doctrine of original antigenic
sin"). The relationship between the various
antigenic components of influenza virus and their
immunogenic response is shown in Table 8. The
HI antibody appears to be the primary immunologic
determinant by inhibiting viral infection of susceptible cells, whereas the neuraminidase antibody is believed to modify the severity of infection by preventing spread of virus to other
target cells. Immunity develops against the
homologous virus and is transient, apparently
because of the localized nature of infection in
the respiratory tract. Moreover, in the case of
influenza A virus, its mutability circumvents
existing immunity and renders the population susceptible to newly emerging virus strains.

4. Pathogenesis. The virus is transmitted by airborne respiratory secretions from infected persons. Following inhalation, the virus multiplies in the ciliated respiratory epithelium, particularly in the nasal and tracheobronchial mucous membranes. In uncomplicated cases, the virus is present in the respiratory secretions 1 to 2 days before and after onset of illness. In complicating influenzal pneumonia, the virus spreads to the bronchiolar and alveolar epithelium, producing foci of infection in the lungs. Although viremia has been occasionally demonstrated, the infection is localized mainly to the respiratory tract and normally does not involve other body organs.

TABLE 8   Major Influenza Virus Antigens

Antigen	Location	Viral Antibody Neutralization	Immunologic Specificity	Serologic Detection
Soluble (S) ribonucleo-protein	Nucleocapsid, also infected cells	–	Type	CF*
Membrane (M) protein	Associated with viral envelope	–	Type	CF
Hemagglu-tinin (H) glycopro-tein	Viral surface	+	Subtype	CF HI** Nt***
Neuramini-dase (N) glycopro-tein	Viral surface	–	Subtype	Neuramini-dase**** inhibition

*Complement fixation
**Hemagglutination inhibition
***Neutralization
****Inhibition of enzymatic release of N-acetyl neuraminic acid from glyoprotein substrate.

5. *Pathology*. Pathologically, influenza
manifests itself as an acute inflammatory reaction in the nasopharyngeal and tracheobronchial
ciliated epithelium with congestion, edema,
necrosis and desquamation of the mucosal epithelial cells. Metaplasia frequently occurs with
regeneration and repair of the respiratory
epithelium. In fatal cases, a hemorrhagic bronchopneumonia is produced in which a mononuclear
cell infiltrate is found in the interstitial
areas with necrosis of the bronchiolar and alveolar epithelium and alveolar capillary throm-
bosis. The lung pathology is often obscured by
a superimposing purulent bacterial pneumonia.

C. DIAGNOSIS.
1. *Clinical*. In epidemic situations, the
abrupt onset of illness and the acute signs and
symptoms of influenza are sufficiently characteristic so that a diagnosis can be made on the
basis of epidemiologic information and clinical
findings. However, in sporadic cases, it is
impossible to make an exact diagnosis without
corroborative virologic studies.
2. *Laboratory*.
a. Isolation of the Virus. Throat or
nasopharyngeal swabs or washings should be collected within 3 days after onset of illness.
The swab specimen is more conveniently taken and
should be placed directly into the transport
medium (tryptose phosphate broth with 0.5 percent gelatin). In fatal influenzal pneumonia,
specimens of lung tissue and tracheal mucosa
should be submitted for viral isolation studies.
Clinical and autopsy specimens must be sent to
the laboratory immediately after collection. If
this is not possible, the specimens should be
stored at -70°C until used. Following receipt
by the laboratory, the specimen is treated with
penicillin and streptomycin and inoculated into
primary monkey kidney cell cultures and/or the
amniotic sac of embryonated chicken eggs. Virus
multiplication is demonstrated by the hemadsorption technique and/or cytopathic effects in the

monkey kidney cells or detection of hemagglutinin
in the egg fluids. Guinea pig, human, or chicken
red blood cells may be used in the hemadsorption
and hemagglutination tests. The virus isolate
is usually identified by the HI test using known
antiserum against current influenza virus strains.
New strains which react poorly, if at all, in the
HI test are further tested by the CF (type- and
strain-specific) and neuraminidase-inhibition
tests for major changes in the hemagglutinin and
neuraminidase antigens. Although neutralization
tests can be performed in cell culture or in
eggs, the procedure is complex and costly and is
not routinely done.

      b. <u>Virus Serology</u>. Acute serum should
be collected immediately after onset of illness
and a convalescent-phase serum about 2 weeks
later. Serum specimens separated from the blood
clot can be stored frozen at $-20^{\circ}C$. The paired
sera are tested simultaneously in the type-
specific complement fixation test using known
influenza type A and B (and C) soluble ribonucleoprotein antigens or in the strain-specific HI
test with selected current virus strains. A
fourfold or greater increase in antibody titer
between the acute and convalescent-phase serums
is significant of recent infection.

D. TREATMENT. There is no specific treatment
for influenza once the disease develops. Supportive therapy, such as bed rest and aspirin
for fever and minor pains, is generally in order.
In the aged, secondary bacterial pulmonary infections present a common problem but once the
specific bacterium is identified effective antibiotic treatment can be initiated. In pregnancy,
respiratory complications may occur and these
must be treated on a supportive and restorative
basis.

E. EPIDEMIOLOGY. The largest pandemic of modern
times occurred in 1918-19 and was almost unques-
tionably due to a particularly virulent strain

of influenza A virus. Since techniques for
influenza virus cultivation were not available
until 1933, isolation of the agent responsible
was not possible and identification studies have
been retrospective based upon influenza antibody
studies. During this pandemic it has been estimated that there were over a billion cases and
in excess of 20 million deaths. It differed
from more recent pandemics in that there was a
high incidence of death due to pulmonary complications in the 20 to 40 year age group. The
mortality was also higher in the aged, and the
number of persons infected was unusually large.
There is great concern among world health officials in regard to the virulence of new antigenic subtypes of influenza A which arise during
the 2 to 3 year cycles. Present day preventive
and control measures may not be sufficient to
materially reduce the devastating effect of a
highly virulent virus on mankind. These measures
would consist of vaccination with existing vaccines which rely on "antigen overlap," or possibly the use of amantadine. There would be a
"lead time" of 4 to 6 months before an adequate
safety-tested supply of vaccine could be produced using an isolate from a current epidemic.
Secondary bacterial infections could, of course,
be controlled by antibiotics. The reality of
the situation becomes apparent when one consid-
ers that in the 1968 epidemic of influenza A in
the United States, there were an estimated 30 million cases and an increase of about 19,000 pneu-
monia-influenza deaths over the normal expected
seasonal number.

      The virus is spread person to person by way
of airborne respiratory tract secretions. The
period of infectivity is from 1 to 2 days before,
until 1 to 2 days after the appearance of signs
and symptoms. The main incidence is in late
fall, winter and early spring, with the largest
number of cases seen in children and young
adults. The disease is rare in infants under one
year of age and has a low attack rate in the aged.
The mortality is, however, highest in the latter
group.

Influenza A occurs in 2 to 3 year cycles and is responsible for the major pandemics. Influenza B is seen at 4 to 6 year intervals in more "localized" epidemics and often as sporadic cases during type A epidemics. Influenza C does not occur in epidemic proportions and produces a mild, often subclinical infection. The apparent short immunity to influenza A and B is misleading, for reinfection during each epidemic is in reality due to antigenic shift or drift of the virus, and not to lack of persistence of protective antibody. This type of mutation accounts for the ability of the virus to overcome preexisting immunity to previously epidemic subtypes. As an individual ages, the number of subtypes to which he has been exposed increases and his influenza antibody mosaic broadens, thus protecting him, at least partially, against new subtypes. This would account for the decreased incidence of the disease in old age. The mechanism by which the virus mutates is not known, but it may involve recombination between subtypes or antigenic alteration due to the level of influenza antibodies present in the host population.

There are a small number of cases which exist worldwide throughout the year. Sporadic cases probably occur until a mutant arises which is sufficiently antigenically different from those to which large segments of the population have been previously exposed, at which time the disease could reach epidemic proportions.

F.   PREVENTION.
     1.   *Artificial Passive Protection*. Passive protection against influenza is not practiced.
     2.   *Artificial Active Immunization*.
          a.   Properties of the Vaccine. The influenza vaccine licensed in the United States is a formaldehyde-inactivated preparation grown in the allantoic cavity of embryonated chicken eggs. The virus is purified by zonal-ultracentrifugation prior to inactivation. The vaccine for use in 1974-75 contains not less than

1200 chick red blood cell agglutinating (CCA)
units of antigen in the following proportions:
700 CCA units of type A/Port Chalmers/1/73 (H_3N_2)
and 500 CCA units of type B/Hong Kong/5/72. The
official name is Influenza Virus Vaccine, Biva-
lent. The vaccine formulation is reviewed at
regular intervals and its makeup changed when
indicated. The philosophy behind its use involves the supposition that the strain of virus
in the current epidemic will be sufficiently antigenically related to that incorporated in the vaccine to confer protection on the vaccinee. If a
major antigenic shift does not occur, the vaccine
efficiency is 40 to 80 percent. The immunity
induced, however, is short (about 6 months).
Live attenuated virus vaccines are under study.

    3. _General Recommendations_. Annual influenza
vaccination is recommended for persons of all ages
who have: heart disease, particularly with mitral
stenosis or cardiac insufficiency, chronic bron-
chopulmonary diseases such as asthma, chronic
bronchitis, bronchiectasis and emphysema, chronic
renal disease and diabetes mellitus and other
chronic metabolic diseases. It is also recommended for older persons, particularly those over 65.*
Persons who provide essential community services
and hospital personnel are also logical candidates for vaccination. Widespread use of the vaccine in the general "healthy" population is not
recommended. Pregnancy is also not considered
a contraindication for vaccination.

    4. _Administration of the Vaccine_. The vac-
cine is given by the subcutaneous route in a
dose recommended on the manufacturer's package
labeling. The new highly purified preparations
require only one inoculation for either primary
or booster vaccination, preferably given by mid-
November.

---

*See Recommendations of the Public Health Service
 Advisory Committee on Immunization Practices--
 Influenza Vaccine. Morbidity and Mortality
 Vol. 23, No. 24, June 15, 1974.

    5. *Side Effects of the Vaccine*. Occasion-
ally there are minor reactions such as low-
grade fever or erythema and tenderness at the
vaccine site.
    6. *Contraindications*. The vaccine contains
small amounts of chicken egg protein and should
not be given to persons who are hypersensitive
to this substance.
    7. *Chemotherapy*. Amantadine hydrochloride
is an orally administered antiviral drug. Its
specificity appears to be limited to certain
influenza A subtypes (Chapter VI). It must be
used with caution in regard to dose level and
in the case of certain underlying diseases
(epilepsy, cerebral arteriosclerosis). It must
also be administered before or shortly after
contact with the virus.

G. CONTROL. There are no specific control
measures other than those given above. Isolation and quarantine of known cases is not effective in stemming an epidemic. Whether or not
amantadine would be effective in controlling an
epidemic would depend upon the type-subtype of
the prevailing virus.

Chapter XIX

MEASLES (RUBEOLA)

A. PROPERTIES OF THE VIRUS. Measles virus contains RNA as its genetic material, has a helical
symmetry, is enveloped and is about 150 nm in
size. It is classified as a member of the paramyxovirus group. It possesses a hemagglutinin
for red blood cells of monkeys and baboons. There
is only one known antigenic type. It is inactivated by 1 percent formaldehyde, ether and 56°C
for 60 minutes. It loses infectivity rapidly at
37°C but remains viable for years when stored at
-70°C.

B. HOST RESPONSE TO INFECTION.
   1. _Incubation_ _Period,_ _Signs_ _and_ _Symptoms_.
The incubation period is 10 to 12 days to onset of
fever. The prodromal syndrome, which lasts about
2 to 3 days, consists of sneezing, nasal discharge, conjunctivitis, photophobia, cough and
fever. Koplik spots, which are considered pathognomonic for measles, appear late in the prodromal
period. They are bilateral small reddish macules
with a bluish-white center which are first seen on
the inner cheek opposite the second molar, spread
to the buccal mucosa, and appear in 90 to 95 percent of all measles cases. The fever and cough
become progressively worse until the appearance
of the rash, about 14 days following initial contact. The rash first appears on the forehead
and behind the ears and subsequently spreads
over the face, neck, trunk and limbs. It is
macular or maculopapular, disappears on pressure,
and may become confluent. After a period of
2 to 3 days the rash begins to disappear in
sequence, with those areas affected first dis-
appearing first. The fever falls coincidentally
with the disappearance of rash. Despite the fact
that measles is a severe disease, most children

recover rapidly. Encephalitis or other residua
may occur in about 1 of every 1000 cases.

    2. *Pathogenesis*. Measles virus enters by
way of the respiratory tract and multiplies in
epithelial cells lining these tissues. It is
also possible that infection can take place
through the eye. The virus also multiplies in
the regional lymphatic tissue and a brief viremia
occurs. After a period of 10 to 11 days, multiplication of the virus is great enough to produce the prodromal signs and symptoms. The virus
becomes widely disseminated by a secondary viremia
at this time, and is present in blood, lung, kidney, spleen, skin, urine and eye secretions.

    3. *Pathology*. The outstanding pathology of
measles is the presence of multinucleated giant
cells which may be found in nasal secretions,
appendix, lymph nodes, tonsils and adenoids. In
encephalitis there are congestion, perivascular
hemorrhage and lymphocytic infiltration. Demyelination occurs later in brain and cord and is
often accompanied by an infiltrate with leukocytes
and monocytes and secondary gliosis.

    4. *Immune Response*. Antibodies against
measles virus can first be detected at the time
of the rash and rise to a peak at about 14 days.
Complement fixing (CF), hemagglutination inhibiting (HI) and virus neutralizing (Nt) antibodies
may be demonstrated. A peculiarity of the immune
response to measles is the persistence of CF antibodies for several years after infection. It is
not uncommon for viral HI and neutralizing antibodies to remain for the lifetime of an individual
but CF antibodies are usually transient. Immunity
is lifetime and second attacks are rare.

    5. *Prognosis*. In well-developed countries
the overall mortality from measles is low, less
than 2 per 100,000 cases. It is higher in children under 4 years of age (about 3 per 100,000)
and lower when contacted later in life (about
1 per 100,000). In West Africa the case fatality
rate may reach a level 200 to 300 times that given
above.

6. *Complications*.

a. <u>Encephalomyelitis</u>. This complication, which occurs 5 to 7 days after the rash, has an incidence of from 1 to 10 cases per 10,000 measles cases. The incidence varies depending upon the epidemic and geographical location. The mortality is about 10 percent, and permanent brain damage and mental retardation may be as high as 65 percent.

b. <u>Otitis Media</u>. Inflammation of the ear is a frequent complication of measles and is usually due to secondary bacterial invasion.

c. <u>Bronchopneumonia</u>. This complication is due to secondary bacterial invasion usually by pneumococci, beta hemolytic streptococci or staphylococci. Measles virus *per se* may produce a frequently fatal "giant-cell" pneumonia (Hecht's pneumonia).

d. <u>Subacute Sclerosing Panencephalitis</u> (SSPE). Present evidence indicates that the progressive neurological deterioration seen in SSPE may be a consequence of persistent measles virus infection. Measles virus has been demonstrated in these patients by cocultivation of brain tissue with African green monkey kidney or HeLa cell cultures. This disease is characterized by progressive mental and motor degeneration. At autopsy, parenchymatous lesions and demyelination are found in both gray and white matter of the brain. Other brain pathology is similar to that of measles encephalitis.

e. <u>Congenital Effects</u>. Since a viremia occurs with measles there is a potential hazard to the fetus. In actual practice, however, it has been found that even if infection occurs in the first trimester of pregnancy the incidence of malformations and fetal death due to measles is low to non-existent.

C. DIAGNOSIS.

1. *Clinical*. Clinical diagnosis is made on the basis of the location, appearance and spread of the rash along with a history and presenting

signs and symptoms. Koplik spots, as previously
described, are considered pathognomonic of measles. They are present in 95 percent of the
cases.
     2. _Laboratory_.
          a. Virus Isolation. Measles virus is
isolated with difficulty _in vitro_ but can be
propagated in a wide variety of human and animal
cell cultures (heart, amnion, kidney). The tissue culture cells of choice are primary human
embryonic or monkey kidney cells. In culture
the virus produces a syncytium or multinucleated
giant cells. Eosinophilic cytoplasmic and nuclear inclusions are present. Measles virus can
be differentiated from other paramyxoviruses by
its ability to hemadsorb monkey red blood cells.
Definitive identification of viral isolates is
based on neutralization or immunofluorescence
tests.
          b. Specimens for Virus Isolation.
          1) Blood--the virus may be isolated
from the blood from slightly before until about
two days after the rash appears.
          2) Nasopharynx--the virus is present
in the nasopharynx during the prodromal stage
until about 48 hours after the appearance of the
rash. It is possible to make a presumptive diagnosis of measles during the prodromal stage by
demonstrating the presence of characteristic multinucleated giant cells (Warthin-Finkeldey cells) in
smears of nasal mucosa. The application of direct
immunofluorescence greatly enhances the sensitivity
of viral detection.
          3) Urine--virus may be isolated from
the urine from the prodromal stage until about
7 days after the appearance of the rash.
          c. Serology. Antibodies first develop
about the time of the onset of the rash and peak
10 to 14 days later. Three types of tests for
their detection are available.
          1) Complement fixation
          2) Neutralization
          3) Hemagglutination inhibition

As with all acute and convalescent serum
serology, a fourfold or greater increase in
antibody titer is required for diagnosis. Patients with SSPE have an elevated CSF and serum
measles antibody.

D.   TREATMENT. There is no specific treatment
for measles. Aspirin and bed rest may be recommended during the febrile period. Antibiotics
are prescribed only in the case of known secondary
bacterial infections.

E.   EPIDEMIOLOGY.
     1.   _Transmission_. The virus is transmitted
by direct contact between an infected and a susceptible person. There are no carriers. The
patient is contagious from the beginning of the
acute stage until about 48 to 72 hours following
the onset of the rash. The major spread is by
secretions of the upper respiratory tract and
nasopharynx. Measles is a highly communicable
disease and is worldwide in distribution. In
urban areas, prior to the use of vaccination,
most children acquired it during the first decade
of life. Approximately 80 to 85 percent of an
urban population at age 20 years can be shown to
have measles antibodies due to a natural infection.
     2.   _Seasonal and Epidemic Incidence_. The
largest number of cases of measles in temperate
zones occur in late winter and early spring; and
epidemics appear every 2 to 3 years.

F.   PREVENTION.
     1.   _Artificial Passive Immunization_. Tempo-
rary protection against measles is possible by
the use of pooled human gamma globulin. The
measles antibody content of such pools is sufficient to prevent the disease if given within
5 days after exposure. The half-life of administered gamma globulin is about 3 weeks, and
complete immunity produced by passive immunization rarely extends beyond a month. The exact
duration depends, of course, on the antibody

content of the gamma globulin. Two preparations
are available, measles immune globulin (MIG) and
immune serum globulin (ISG). They are prepared
by cold alcohol fractionation of pools of human
blood plasma and contain 16.5 percent total protein. It must be remembered that all types of
antibody present in the serum of the persons from
whom the plasma was collected will be contained
in the gamma globulin. The dose level with
either preparation is 0.1 ml per pound of body
weight.

    2. _Artificial_ _Active_ _Immunity_.

      a. <u>Measles Virus Vaccines</u>. There are
several licensed measles vaccines; all consist
of live attenuated measles virus produced _in vitro_
in cultures of either chick embryo or canine kidney cells. The main difference between them lies
in the degree of attenuation and thus the clinical response. The Edmonston B attenuated strain
produces rectal temperatures of from 100 to 103°F
in 30 percent of the vaccinees.

    The fever usually begins about the 6th
day after vaccination and lasts 5 days. The incidence can be reduced to 15 percent by the simultaneous administration of 0.01 ml per pound of
body weight of MIG or ISG at a different inoculation site. A separate syringe should be used.
The further attenuated vaccines (Schwarz and
Attenuvax) produce the same high fever in 15 percent of the recipients. It is _not_ recommended
that MIG or ISG be given with these further attenuated vaccines. It is interesting to note
that in spite of the high fever these children
have relatively little discomfort. The mild or
inapparent disease induced is noncommunicable.
These vaccines are all highly efficient and
result in a seroconversion of about 95 percent.
The duration of immunity is at least 10 years
and may well be lifetime.

      b. <u>Vaccine Usage</u>.

      1) General recommendations--all
susceptible children should be vaccinated at
about one year of age. Infants of 9 to 12 months
may be vaccinated, but the number of seroconver-

sions will be reduced owing to maternal antibody.
Vaccination of adults is seldom necessary since
most Americans over 15 years of age have a natural active immunity due to previous infection
with measles.

        2) Dose--a single subcutaneous in-
oculation is given. No booster is necessary.
If the Edmonston B strain is used, it should be
accompanied by MIG, 0.01 ml per pound of body
weight, given in a separate syringe at a different site.

        3) Revaccination--children under
the age of 9 months who have been vaccinated
with virus and MIG should be revaccinated with
live virus vaccine. Children who have previously been given the inactivated measles vaccine
should,regardless of their age at the time of
administration, also be revaccinated with live
virus vaccine.

        4) Use of vaccine following mea-
sles exposure--if administered before or within
two days of exposure, live measles vaccine will
prevent the disease.

        5) Contraindications--measles vac-
cine should not be administered in cases of
leukemia or during periods of lowered resistance
due to therapy with steroids, alkylating agents,
radiation or under other conditions where the
immune response is depressed. It should also
not be administered during pregnancy or in the
presence of a febrile disease.

G. CONTROL. Patients should be isolated from
the time of first diagnosis until 2 to 3 days
after the appearance of the rash. Vaccination
is a highly effective control method.

Chapter XX

MUMPS

A. PROPERTIES OF THE VIRUS. Mumps virus contains RNA as its genetic material, is about 100
to 200 nm in size, has a helical capsid symmetry,
is enveloped and possesses a hemagglutinin for
chicken, human O and guinea pig red blood cells.
It is classified as a paramyxovirus and only one
antigenic type exists. The virus has two distinct identifiable antigens, the V (viral) antigen associated with the hemagglutinin which gives
rise to protective antibodies, and the S (soluble)
antigen which is associated with the nucleocapsid.
The virus also contains a neuraminidase. The infective particle is inactivated by ether, chloroform, formalin, $56^{\circ}C$ for 20 minutes, ultraviolet
light and drying. It remains viable for years
when stored at $-70^{\circ}C$.

B. HOST RESPONSE TO INFECTION.
   1. Incubation Period, Signs and Symptoms.
The incubation period of mumps is usually 18 to
21 days, with a range of 14 to 28 days. There is
normally a slight fever, headache and malaise pri-
or to the swelling of the parotid gland. The enlargement may remain unilateral, but often becomes
bilateral 1 to 5 days after the first gland is
affected. Swelling reaches a maximum in 2 days,
persists for 7 to 10 days, and disappears without
sequelae. About one in five of all males over
the age of 13 develops orchitis 1 to 7 days following the parotid gland inflammation. Sterility
does not usually result owing to the fact that
only about 15 percent of the cases are bilateral,
and even then not all glandular tissue is involved.
Complete recovery usually takes place within two
weeks. Aseptic meningitis, which develops about
a week after the parotid gland swelling, is another complication of mumps. It has an incidence
of 1 to 10 percent of all cases, and is usually

mild and self-resolving.

2. _Pathogenesis_. The mumps virus reaches the salivary glands by one of two possible pathways: a) the virus enters by way of the respiratory tract, where it multiplies in this tissue and the local lymph nodes, resulting in a viremia and infection of the salivary glands; b) the virus reaches the salivary glands directly from the mouth by way of the salivary ducts, resulting in virus growth and a viremia. In either case other organs, testes, ovaries or central nervous system may be infected following the viremia.

3. _Pathology_. In those few cases where mumps pathology has been studied it has been found that the cells of the ducts of the salivary glands show evidence of destruction and infiltration with leucocytes. In severe orchitis there is a degeneration of the epithelium of the seminiferous tubules and small areas of hemorrhage in the testes. In the pancreas there is interstitial edema, fat necrosis and degeneration of the islets of Langerhans.

4. _Immune Response_. Soluble (S) complement fixing antibodies appear 7 to 10 days following onset of symptoms, rise to a maximum at about 4 weeks and decline rapidly. Viral (V) complement fixing and hemagglutinin inhibiting and neutralizing antibodies are best determined about 14 days after onset and are detectable for several years. Immunity is lifelong and second attacks are rare.

5. _Prognosis_. Complete recovery occurs in uncomplicated mumps cases. Severe orchitis may result in a reduced sperm count but sterility is rare. Meningoencephalitis is normally mild and resolves with no sequelae. Deafness is a major though rare complication. There are no definite data on effect on the fetus of mumps acquired during pregnancy.

C. DIAGNOSIS.

1. _Clinical_. A febrile episode followed by parotid swelling either unilateral or bilateral

establishes a clinical diagnosis with reasonable
accuracy. This is particularly true in epidemics.
Isolated cases are more difficult to diagnose and
other nonspecific causes of salivary gland enlargement such as neoplasm or duct blockage must
be considered. Positive diagnosis can only be
established through laboratory procedures. These
tests are particularly helpful when mumps meningitis occurs without parotid involvement.

    2. _Laboratory_.

       a. <u>Isolation of the Virus</u>. The virus is
present in the saliva and urine for up to 4 to
5 days after disease onset. In mumps meningitis
it is present during the same period in the spinal
fluid. Isolation may be carried out by amniotic
cavity inoculation of 8-day-old chick embryos or
in primary monkey kidney or human embryonic
kidney or lung tissue cultures. Identification
is made by specific mumps hemadsorption-inhibition or neutralization. Specimens should be
stored frozen if not used within a few hours of
collection.

       b. <u>Serology</u>. The most commonly employed
test is complement fixation. Hemagglutinin inhibition is less reliable owing to cross reactions
with parainfluenza viruses. Serum is collected
shortly after onset and 10 to 14 days later. The
tests are run with specific mumps antigen and a
fourfold increase in antibody titer is diagnostic.
A presumptive diagnosis may be made using a single
acute serum specimen collected within a few days
after disease onset. This is based on the fact
that S complement fixing antibodies develop early
and V complement fixing antibodies develop somewhat later. Thus, if the CF test is run with S
and V antigen and the S titer is elevated with
lower or no detectable V, it indicates a current
infection. Both S and V titer are elevated in a
recent infection.

D. TREATMENT. There is no specific therapy for
mumps. In most cases the disease is mild and
treatment is symptomatic (headache, fever). Surgical intervention to relieve pressure due to
edema may be necessary in severe orchitis.

E. EPIDEMIOLOGY. Mumps is spread through saliva by direct contact, fomites or aerosols. The
virus is present in the oral cavity from 6 days
before until 9 days after the parotid swelling.
It is most prevalent in late winter or early
spring in the 5 to 15 year age group. Epidemics
occur every 7 to 8 years and the disease is
worldwide in distribution. As many as 30 percent of all cases are subclinical. Eighty to
90 percent of the adult population is immune by
virtue of contact with the virus. In the first
22 weeks of 1974 there were 35,645 reported cases
of mumps in the United States.

F. PREVENTION.
    1. _Artificial_ _Active_ _Immunity_. The mumps
vaccine is composed of live attenuated virus grown
on chick embryo cell cultures. It produces an inapparent noncommunicable infection with 95 percent
antibody conversion in recipients. It is given
as a single subcutaneous inoculation in the volume
specified by the manufacturer. No booster dose
is needed. It is recommended at any age after
1 year, but should not be used prior to this time
owing to interference by maternal antibody. Immunity is known to last at least 6 years. The vaccine is contraindicated in pregnancy, immunosuppressive therapy, severe febrile illness, general
malignancies or known hypersensitivity to chicken
egg protein.
    2. _Artificial_ _Passive_ _Immunization_. Pas-
sive immunization with pooled human gamma globulin
is not practical owing to the low mumps antibody
titer in adults. Mumps convalescent serum gamma
globulin has been given shortly after exposure
to prevent the disease in male adults where orchitis is a complication and in other cases where
mumps vaccination is contraindicated.

G. CONTROL. Active immunization is the only
method of controlling mumps. Isolation of cases
is not a practical solution since there are at
least 30 percent subclinical cases and the disease may be spread 6 days prior to the onset of
symptoms.

Chapter XXI

PARAINFLUENZA VIRUSES (TYPES 1, 2, 3, 4)

A. PROPERTIES OF THE VIRUSES. These viruses contain RNA as their genetic material, are approximately 150 to 250 nm in size, have a helical
symmetry and possess a lipoprotein envelope. They
also have the property of agglutinating human,
chicken or guinea pig red blood cells. The hemagglutinin spikes project from the envelope which
also contains the neuraminidase. Four antigenic
types have been recognized on the basis of complement fixation (CF), hemagglutination inhibition (HI) and neutralization (Nt). In addition,
Type 4 has two subtypes A and B. There is no
common group antigen but the viruses share minor
related antigens. An immunological relationship
exists between mumps virus and parainfluenza
viruses so that a heterotypic antibody response
occurs in individuals who have had a prior infection with any of these viruses. Antibody response
to a primary infection is, of course, type specific. The parainfluenza viruses are classified as
members of the paramyxovirus group. Infectivity
of these viruses is rapidly lost at temperatures
of 37°C or higher. They are also inactivated by
ether, chloroform or other lipid solvents as well
as common disinfectants. They may be stored for
years at -70°C if 5 percent chicken or bovine
serum is added to the suspending medium.

B. HOST RESPONSE TO INFECTION.
    1. _Incubation Period, Signs and Symptoms_.
The incubation period is 2 to 6 days depending
upon the virus type involved. Disease syndromes
reported in humans are upper respiratory tract
infections (types 1, 3, and 4), bronchitis and
bronchopneumonia (types 1 and 3), and croup
(types 1 and 2). The disease is more severe in
infants and children than in adults.

2. *Pathogenesis*. The virus enters by the respiratory route and multiplies in the epithelial cells of the upper respiratory tract. It is normally confined to this area, but in infants and young children it may also invade the larynx, trachea, bronchi, bronchioles, and lungs. Thus, the results of the more severe infection may be bronchopneumonia, obstruction of the airway, or laryngotracheobronchitis. Although a viremia probably occurs, it has not been demonstrated.

3. *Pathology*. The number of cases coming to autopsy has been too few in number to allow a definitive pathological picture to be described.

4. *Immune Response*. Infection with parainfluenza viruses gives rise to the production of CF, HI and Nt antibodies. In primary infections antibodies are first detectable at 5 to 7 days and peak at about 2 weeks. Heterotypic antibodies are formed when infection with any of the parainfluenza viruses or mumps follows a prior infection with one of these viruses. Reinfection also takes place, but its frequency is not known. The severity of the disease due to these viruses is lessened when the individual has had a prior exposure to a homo- or heterotypic parainfluenza virus. Resistance to infection *per se* appears to be more related to secretory IgA than to IgG. It is probably for this reason that maternally acquired antibody does not protect the newborn.

5. *Prognosis*. Infection in older children and adults results in a mild self-resolving disease. In infants and young children the disease is more severe and may require hospitalization. The mortality with proper supportive treatment is low and complete recovery is the rule.

C. DIAGNOSIS.

1. *Clinical*. There are no outstanding clinical characteristics of parainfluenza virus infections that are of value in establishing these viruses as the causative agents of a given disease. However, the high frequency with which they cause croup, bronchitis and bronchopneumonia in early infancy necessitates that they be included in a differential diagnosis of these conditions.

2.   _Laboratory_.
       a.   Isolation of the Virus. Nasopharyn-
geal and oropharyngeal swabs are the specimens
of choice for virus isolation.   The best substrate for the isolation of parainfluenza viruses
is either primary monkey or human cell cultures.
Cytopathic changes, which are not easily discernible, occur with type 2 virus only and consist
of syncytia formation in the cultures.   Eosinophilic cytoplasmic inclusions are also found in
H & E stained cultures.   The presence of virus
in the cultures may be detected in the absence
of cell changes by adding guinea pig erythrocytes
to the cell sheet.   In the presence of parainfluenza virus, the red cells are adsorbed to the
cell sheet (hemadsorption).   This test is not
specific for parainfluenza since other hemagglutinating viruses may be capable of the same response.   Identification of suspected isolates
is accomplished by hemadsorption inhibition or
HI.   Specific antiserum is prepared by immunizing
hamsters or guinea pigs with each type of virus.
The subtypes A and B of type 4 virus can only
be identified by neutralization.
       b.   Serology. Acute serum collected in
the first few days of disease and convalescent
serum collected about 2 weeks later are used to
detect a rise in CF, or HI antibodies.   A standard fourfold or greater increase is considered
diagnostic.   The test most commonly employed is
CF.   The specific type of parainfluenza virus
involved can only be determined by comparative
serological testing because of the heterotypic
antibodies which are produced.   The greatest rise
in antibody occurs against the specific virus involved.

D.   TREATMENT.   There is no specific treatment
for parainfluenza viruses.

E.   EPIDEMIOLOGY.   The portal of entry is the
respiratory tract.   Limited epidemics have been
reported with type 3 and this type has been shown
to spread with great efficiency in closed nonimmune populations.   The disease is worldwide

in distribution and most cases occur in late fall
or early winter. Infection with type 3 is acquired early in life: by age 1 year about 50 percent and by age 6 years most of the children in
the United States have antibodies to this type.
Infection with types 1, 2, and 4 takes place
slightly later in life and by age 10 years about
75 percent of all children can be shown to have
antibodies to these types. Type 4 often causes
subclinical or very mild infections. Reinfection
with a homologous type takes place, and it is
doubtful if specific immunity lasts much more
than a year.

F.   PREVENTION.
     1. *Artificial Passive Immunization*. Passive
protection against the parainfluenza viruses is
not practiced.
     2. *Artificial Active Immunization*. There
are no vaccines available for immunization against
parainfluenza viruses. Inactivated vaccines for
types 1, 2, and 3 have been tested in infants
and shown to produce serum neutralizing antibodies
but not IgA. Since IgA plays an important part
in preventing infection with respiratory viruses,
it may be necessary to develop a live attenuated
respiratory tract administered vaccine before they
can be controlled.

G.   CONTROL.   There are no specific control methods
for parainfluenza virus infections.

Chapter XXII

RESPIRATORY SYNCYTIAL VIRUS

A. PROPERTIES OF THE VIRUS. Respiratory syncytial virus (RSV) contains RNA as its genetic
material, is approximately 100 to 140 nm in size,
has a helical symmetry and possesses an envelope.
It is the only member of the paramyxovirus group
for which a hemagglutinin has not been demonstrated. The virus is extremely labile and is
rapidly inactivated at either room or refrigerator temperature. It remains viable for several
days when frozen at -10 to -30°C. The stability
may be increased to several months by adding
10 percent protein (such as serum) to the suspending solution prior to rapid freezing and storing
at -70°C. Destruction of the envelope with ether
or chloroform results in inactivation of the virus.

B. HOST RESPONSE TO INFECTION.
1. *Incubation Period, Signs and Symptoms*.
The incubation period of RSV is 4 to 5 days. The
disease most often affects infants in the first
4 to 6 months of life. Signs and symptoms are fever, exudative or erythematous pharyngitis, bronchiolitis, bronchopneumonia, or croup. Examination by X-ray may show interstitial pneumopathy
with emphysema. The disease usually resolves
spontaneously within a week or 10 days, but fatal
cases have been reported in infants. Primary infection or reinfection in older children and adults
normally results in mild upper respiratory tract
symptoms.
2. *Pathogenesis*. The virus enters by way of
the respiratory tract and multiples in the epithelial cells in this area. In older children and
adults the virus is limited to growth in the upper
respiratory tract. In infants it may spread to
the bronchi, bronchioli or pulmonary parenchyma.
3. *Pathology*. Those few cases which have
come to autopsy have shown an interstitial pneu-

monia consisting of a mononuclear infiltrate and
necrotizing lesions of the epithelium of the
bronchi and bronchioles.

　　4. _Immune Response_. Complement fixing and
neutralizing antibodies are first detectable
about 5 days after the appearance of clinical
signs and symptoms and peak at about 2 weeks.
In infants less than 7 months of age, the response in the case of both CF and Nt antibodies
is poor and occurs in less than 50 percent of
all cases.

　　5. _Prognosis_. The disease in older children
and adults is mild and cures spontaneously without complications. In infants, even though the
virus can cause a severe bronchopneumonia often
requiring hospitalization, fatal cases are rare
and complete recovery in 1 to 3 weeks is the
rule.

C. DIAGNOSIS.

　　1. _Clinical_. As is the case with most virus
diseases, exact clinical diagnosis of the agent
responsible is impossible. However, RSV should
be suspected in all cases of bronchopneumonia or
bronchiolitis in infants less than 6 months of
age. It is the most common cause of bronchiolitis in infants. Diagnosis may be aided further
by knowledge of an ongoing epidemic.

　　2. _Laboratory_.

　　　　a. Isolation of the Virus. The extreme
lability of the virus makes isolation difficult,
and if at all possible, specimens should be inoculated immediately into susceptible tissue
cultures without freezing. If the specimen must
be frozen prior to inoculation, 10 percent bovine
serum or albumin added to a small amount of suspending medium will prolong virus viability.
The virus is present in the nasal and pharyngeal
secretions early in the disease, and may be isolated from swabs taken from these areas. The
substrates most often used are continuous human
cell cultures. (Hep#2, HeLa, WI-38) or primary
human or monkey kidney cell cultures. The
virus produces characteristic multinucleated

giant cells (syncytia), and eosinophilic intracytoplasmic inclusion bodies in 3 to 14 days.
Identification is accomplished by means of CF
or Nt with specific antiserum. Immunofluorescence may also be used for isolate identification
or may be applied directly to exfoliated cells
from the respiratory tract.

       b. _Serology_. The most commonly used
method of laboratory diagnosis of RSV infection
is complement fixation. Neutralization may also
be used, but it is more time consuming and expensive. Acute and convalescent serum should
be collected early in the disease and at 10 to
14 days; a standard fourfold or greater increase in antibody is considered diagnostic.
Both CF and Nt tests are highly efficient (80
to 90 percent) for detecting antibody in the
case of older children and adults, but less efficient in the case of infants less than 7 months
of age.

D. TREATMENT. There is no specific treatment
for RSV infection. Therapy is mainly supportive.

E. EPIDEMIOLOGY. The virus is spread person
to person by means of secretions from the respiratory tract of infected persons. The disease
is worldwide in distribution, and epidemics,
mainly in infants and young children, occur in
the fall, winter and spring but seldom in summer.
In the United States 30 percent of all infants
by age 1 year, and 95 percent of all children by
age 5 years, show the presence of RSV antibody.
Reinfection in older children and adults can take
place, despite the demonstrated presence of circulating antibody.

F. PREVENTION.
    1. _Artificial Passive Immunization_. Pas-
sive protection is not practiced in the case of
RSV.
    2. _Artificial Active Immunization_. There
is no vaccine available for immunization against
RSV. Formalin-inactivated alum-precipitated

vaccines have been tested in humans and shown to
produce circulating antibody. However, subsequent natural infection with RSV resulted in a
more severe infection than normally occurred
without prior exposure to the vaccine. This may
have been the result of either a hypersensitivity
reaction or an interaction between circulating
antibody and virus on infected cells. Whether
or not live attenuated virus vaccines which might
circumvent this problem can be produced is open
to question and under study.

G.   CONTROL.   There are no specific control methods for RSV infections.

be either abrupt or gradual. The syndrome
sists of fever, headache, malaise, abdominal
a, nausea and stiffness of the neck. There
be muscle weakness and positive Kernig and
dzinski signs can be elicited. Cerebro-
al fluid chemistry shows a normal sugar and
htly increased protein. There may be an
reased cell count, mostly lymphocytes, of 100
00 cells per cubic mm. The condition is seen
ly in children and lasts for several days and
ppears without sequelae. Coxsackieviruses
B1 through 6 and A2, 4, 7, and 9 are most
only involved, but other type A viruses have
implicated.

b. <u>Herpangina</u>. The incubation period of
disease is 7 days or less and begins
ptly with fever, which may reach 104°F, sore
at, nausea, dysphagia and anorexia. Vomit-
and diarrhea may also occur. Four to 6 days
r onset there appear small discrete vesicular
ons on the anterior pillars of the fauces.
are low in number, a few mm in diameter and
ish-white with a red periphery. The lesions
ease in size over the next few days, rupture,
rate and heal. The disease is most often
in young children and, except for convul-
s which may occur owing to the high fever, is
and resolves after 4 to 6 days with no
elae. Coxsackie A viruses are most often
lved.

c. <u>Epidemic Pleurodynia (Devil's Grip,</u>
<u>holm Disease, Epidemic Myalgia)</u>. The incuba-
period is less than a week, probably 3 to
ys. The onset is abrupt with fever (101 to
F), headache, anorexia, sore throat, gastro-
stinal disturbances and a severe pain in the
les of the abdominal wall or intercostal
es. The pain is often so intense as to make
thing difficult. In certain cases the con-
tiva has also been involved. The chest pains
for 2 to 14 days, may recur and usually
lve without any sequelae. The Coxsackieviruses
often involved are types B1 through B6.

Chapter XXIII

COXSACKIEVIRUSES

A. PROPERTIES OF THE VIRUSES. Coxs
contain RNA as their genetic materia
imately 28 nm in diameter, have a cu
hedral symmetry and do not have an e
They are classified, along with the
and polioviruses, as enteroviruses a
of the picornavirus group. Coxsacki
subdivided into type A, which has 23
and type B, which has 6 members. Th
division is based on the response of
mice to inoculation with the virus.
viruses produce a flaccid paralysis
of a diffuse inflammation of the ske
Coxsackie B viruses produce a more f
of skeletal muscle, inflammation of
pads and occasionally pancreatitis,
and myocarditis. Precise identifica
sackievirus type is made by neutral
specific antiserum. There is a subc
complement fixing antigen for Coxsa
which is also shared with A-9. The
of the A subgroups are less commonl
thus more type specific. Certain C
possess a hemagglutinin for human t
cells. The Coxsackieviruses are re
ether, chloroform, lysol and alcohol
inactivated rapidly by formaldehyde
boiling or $60^{o}C$ for 30 minutes. Th
fective for years when stored froze
$-70^{o}C$.

B. HOST RESPONSE TO INFECTION. Al
majority of Coxsackievirus infectio
clinical, they may be associated wi
of clinical syndromes.
    1. _Incubation Period, Signs an_
        a. _Aseptic Meningitis_. Th
period is 2 to 7 days and the onse

may
con
pai
may
Bru
spi
sli
inc
to
mos
dis
typ
com
bee

thi
abr
thr
ing
aft
les
The
gra
inc
ulc
see
sio
mil
seq
inv

Born
tion
7 da
102°
inte
musc
spac
brea
junc
last
reso
most

d. Respiratory Disease. There is increasing evidence that certain of the type A and
B Coxsackieviruses can produce acute upper respiratory diseases and "common colds," and a possible pneumonitis in infants.

e. Neonatal Myocarditis. This rare complication of Coxsackievirus infection is seen in
the first 10 days of life as an acute condition
in which the infant has diarrhea, vomiting followed by difficulty in breathing, tachycardia
and cyanosis. The mortality is quite high (about
50 percent). Recovery may take place with sequelae that are seen later in life. The virus
types most often involved are B1 through B5.

f. Acute Primary Pericarditis. The incubation period is from 2 to 6 days. Epidemics
of this disease have been reported in children
and adults. There are electrocardiographic
abnormalities and retrosternal pain which is
aggravated by movement. Spontaneous resolution
normally occurs within several days. The viruses
most often involved are types B1 through B5.

g. Skin Eruptions. There are a wide
variety of summer febrile illnesses due to any of
several types of Coxsackie A and B virus. Most
are accompanied by a rash which progresses through
a macule-papule-vesicle sequence. As might be
expected these syndromes are often confused with
other childhood diseases such as rubella and
chickenpox. One highly specific response is that
of "hand, foot and mouth disease," most often due
to type A16, and less frequently types 5 and 10.
In this case there are vesicular lesions in the
oral cavity (oropharynx, buccal mucosa and tongue)
and on the dorsal surface of the hands and feet.
Cutaneous manifestations in all cases resolve
within 2 to 3 days and there are no sequelae.

2. Pathogenesis. The virus enters the body
through the oral cavity or respiratory tract.
It multiplies in the pharynx and small intestine,
penetrates the blood stream and a viremia ensues.
Dissemination to any of the wide variety of organs
involved takes place, based in part on the predilection of a particular virus type for a

particular tissue. The virus exits by way of the respiratory and alimentary tracts.

3. *Pathology*. The few cases of fatal Cox-sackievirus infections have usually involved neonatal myocarditis. There was an edema, interstitial infiltration of the myocardium by mononuclear cells and necrosis of the myocardial fibers. There was also a diffuse cellular necro-sis of the pancreas, liver, kidney, adrenals and brain.

4. *Immune Response*. Complement fixing, neutralizing, and hemagglutinin inhibiting (where applicable) antibodies are apparent at about a week after onset and peak at about three weeks. Neutralizing antibodies persist in low titer for years, perhaps for life. The CF antibodies de-crease over a period of several months and are difficult to detect after 6 months to a year. Immunity is type-specific and long lasting.

5. *Prognosis*. Coxsackievirus infections are seldom fatal, except in the case of myocar-ditis of the newborn. Recovery from most other Coxsackievirus infections is complete and secon-dary infections are uncommon.

C. DIAGNOSIS.
1. *Clinical*. A presumptive diagnosis may be made in some of the Coxsackievirus syndromes, but confirmation must be made by the laboratory. Acute respiratory disease, summer rashes, and aseptic meningitis may be caused by a wide variety of viruses and defy clinical diagnosis. On the other hand, epidemics of Bornholm disease, acute pericarditis, or hand, foot and mouth disease have signs and symptoms specific enough for a fairly accurate clinical diagnosis.
2. *Laboratory*.
a. Isolation of the Virus. The virus is most easily isolated from the throat in the first few days after onset of illness and from the stool for several weeks thereafter. In cases of aseptic meningitis the virus may also be isolated from the CSF during the acute stage. Intra-cerebral inoculation of newborn mice represents

the only method for the isolation of *all* A and
B types. Tissue cultures of rhesus monkey kidney and human amnion, kidney, WI-38 or HeLa
cells may be used for the isolation of types
B1 through B6. Type A viruses are difficult to
isolate by this technique, except for certain
types which grow readily in HeLa or monkey kidney cells. The cytopathic effect manifested by
Coxsackieviruses consists of cell rounding and
shrinking with nuclear pyknosis and is also
characteristic of other enteroviruses (echo,
polio). Precise identification is made by Nt
tests with specific antiserum.
        b. Serology. Serum should be collected
shortly after onset of illness and 2 to 3 weeks
later. The most commonly used tests are complement fixation and neutralization. The CF antibodies are not type specific and may develop as
a heterotypic response to either type A or B as
a result of a previous infection. Neutralization
is required for specific type identification.
The large number of members in the Coxsackievirus
group makes it unreasonable to carry out serologic
tests for all virus types. Quite often a specific
number of types within a given disease syndrome
will be selectively tested. For example, B1
through B6 could be tested for neutralization in
tissue culture with acute and convalescent serum
from aseptic meningitis or pericarditis cases.
A fourfold or greater increase in antibody titer
is required for diagnosis.

D. TREATMENT. There is no specific treatment
for Coxsackievirus infections. Therapy is symptomatic and usually consists of relieving pain or
fever.

E. EPIDEMIOLOGY. Man is the reservoir for Coxsackieviruses and they are worldwide in distribution. The route of spread is fecal-oral, person
to person by respiratory secretions or by fomites.
It is also possible that flies may spread the
disease from contaminated sewage. The source of
the virus is the throat for up to a few days after
onset, and feces for up to five weeks longer. The

viremia which occurs plays little or no direct role in transmission. Subclinical cases occur. Outbreaks or small epidemics often arise within family groups or in closed institutions. The main seasonal incidence is in the summer and fall.

F. PREVENTION. There are no vaccines available for the prevention of Coxsackievirus infections.

G. CONTROL. There are no specific control measures. As is the case with all suspected or diagnosed virus diseases, contact of neonates with infected persons should be avoided.

Chapter XXIV

ECHOVIRUSES (E.C.H.O.)

A. PROPERTIES OF THE VIRUS. Echoviruses
(Enteric Cytopathic Human Orphan Viruses) contain RNA as their genetic material, are 24 to 30
nm in diameter, have a cubic icosahedral symmetry and do not possess an envelope. Thirty-
four types were originally classified but subsequently it was found that types 10, 28 and
34 were members of other virus groups. Thus,
there are presently 31 types, with numbers 10 and
28 being left unassigned. They are classified as
enteroviruses in the picornavirus group. Unlike
Coxsackieviruses they do not produce disease when
inoculated into suckling mice. Complement fixing
antigens tend to be type-specific but occasionally
cross-react with other echovirus members. Types
3, 6, 7, 11, 12, 13, 19, 20, 21, 24, 29, 30 and
33 have a hemagglutinin for human group O red
blood cells. The echoviruses are resistant to
ether, chloroform and alcohol. They are inactivated by 1 percent formaldehyde and boiling. They
remain viable for weeks in water and sewage and
may be stored effectively for years at -20 to
-70°C.

B. HOST RESPONSE TO INFECTION.
  1. _Incubation Period, Signs and Symptoms_.
      a. _Aseptic Meningitis_. The incubation
period is usually 3 to 5 days. The onset is
abrupt with fever, headache, nuchal rigidity,
nausea, sore throat and muscle pain. The CSF is
clear and a lymphocytic pleocytosis is evident.
A maculopapular rash often accompanies the
disease but its nature and presence depend upon
the echovirus type involved. It is present on the
face, neck, trunk, thorax and extremities as small
pale red lesions 1 to 4 mm in diameter. It is
most prominent in children when the infection is
due to echovirus type 9. There may be muscle

weakness present for a few days but it is self-
resolving without sequelae. Epidemics of echovirus meningitis are mainly caused by types 9,
4, 6, 30 and, occasionally, by types 11, 14, 16
and 19. Many other types may be involved in sporadic cases. A small number of cases may develop
an encephalitis and paralysis.

      b. <u>Boston Exanthem Disease</u>. This disease
was first reported in 1951 in Boston, Massachusett
Two distinct syndromes were reported, both due to
echovirus 16. The Boston exanthem *per se* involved
a maculopapular rash and signs and symptoms similar to those reported for aseptic meningitis abov
but with no meningitis. The second syndrome con-
sisted of meningitis without rash. Epidemics
have been reported among children and adults from
several other cities. It is highly contagious,
occurs mainly in the summer and recovery is complete.

      c. <u>Respiratory Disease</u>. Several echo-
viruses may play a role in mild febrile upper
respiratory infections and influenza-like illnesse

      d. <u>Gastroenteritis</u>. A large number of the
echoviruses can cause outbreaks of diarrhea and
intestinal upset in adults, children and infants.
In infants the condition can be severe, with blood
watery stools and dehydration.

    2. *Pathogenesis*. The virus enters the body
by way of the oral cavity or respiratory tract,
multiplies in the pharynx, tonsils and small intestine and is excreted in the feces and respiratory secretions. The virus may penetrate the intestine and produce a viremia which leads to the
infection of other organs. In meningitis the rout
of the virus to the meninges is not known. In man
cases the virus does not penetrate beyond the primary tissue infected.

    3. *Pathology*. The echoviruses produce nonfat
diseases and the pathology of those few cases comi
to autopsy is not well defined.

    4. *Immune Response*. Complement fixing (CF),
neutralizing (Nt) and hemagglutination inhibiting
(HI) (where applicable) antibodies are detectable
about a week after disease onset and peak at about

2 to 3 weeks. Neutralizing and HI antibodies persist in low titer for years, perhaps lifetime.
Complement fixing antibodies cannot be detected
after a period less than a year.

   5. *Prognosis*. The outcome of echovirus infection is highly favorable. Meningitis is self-
resolving without sequelae and only an occasional
fatal case has been reported. Dehydration can
be a problem in infants with diarrhea. Secondary
bacterial complications are uncommon.

C. DIAGNOSIS.
   1. *Clinical*. As with most instances where
a virus group is responsible for a wide variety
of disease syndromes, a clinical diagnosis can
at best be only presumptive. In the case of
aseptic meningitis, with or without rash, echoviruses should be considered in the differential
diagnosis. In outbreaks or epidemics of diarrhea
or rash (such as Boston exanthem), these viruses
must also be considered as etiological agents.
Signs and symptoms alone are not characteristic
enough to establish an exact diagnosis. This can
only be done in cooperation with the laboratory.
   2. *Laboratory*.
       a. Isolation of the Viruses. The viruses
may be isolated from the throat from onset of
illness until several days later, and are present
in stools for several weeks. In meningitis, virus
is present in the cerebrospinal fluid during the
acute stage. Cell cultures of rhesus monkey and
human kidneys as well as human lung (WI-38) support the growth of all known echoviruses, producing a characteristic "enterovirus" CPE. Identification is made by neutralization with type-
specific antiserum.
       b. Serology. The large number of echo-
viruses which may be involved in a variety of
disease syndromes makes serological studies using
acute and convalescent serum impractical. As
with Coxsackieviruses, quite often a number of
"most likely" candidates in a specific disease
or preferably a virus isolated from the patient
may be run. When studies are done, neutraliza-

tion with specific type echovirus is the test of
choice, and serum collected at disease onset or
shortly thereafter and at 2 to 3 weeks is required. A standard fourfold or greater increase
in antibody level is required for diagnosis.

D.   TREATMENT. There is no specific treatment.
Therapy is symptomatic and supportive.

E.   EPIDEMIOLOGY. Echovirus-related diseases
are worldwide in distribution, are prevalent in
the summer and fall, more common in children
than in adults, and have a slightly higher incidence in males than in females. The majority
of the infections are subclinical and they can
often be isolated from stools of healthy individuals. They are transmitted by the fecal-oral or
respiratory route or by contaminated fomites or
food. Insects have not been directly implicated
in their transmission. They remain viable for
long periods in water and sewage, and thus could
be spread in this manner.

F.   PREVENTION.
     1. _Active_ _Immunization_. There are no vac-
cines available for echoviruses.
     2. _Passive_ _Immunization_. Passive protection
is not practiced in the case of echoviruses.
Transplacental passage of maternal antibodies has
been shown.

G.   CONTROL. There are no specific control
measures.

Chapter XXV

POLIOVIRUSES

A. PROPERTIES OF THE VIRUSES. The viruses of
poliomyelitis contain RNA as their genetic material, have cubic icosahedral symmetry, are about
30 nm in diameter and nonenveloped. They are
classified as enteroviruses in the picornavirus
group and three distinct types, 1, 2 and 3, are
known. They retain their infectivity for long
periods in water, sewage, milk and foods. They
are inactivated by drying, pasteurization, boiling, chlorine (0.1 ppm) and formalin. They are
not inactivated by ether, chloroform, alcohol
and most common disinfectants. They remain
viable for years when stored frozen.

B. HOST RESPONSE TO INFECTION.
    1. _Incubation Period, Signs and Symptoms_.
The incubation period is about 10 days with ex-
tremes of 3 to 30 days. In 90 to 95 percent of
the cases the disease is mild and characterized
by low-grade fever, constipation, headache,
nausea, sore throat or vomiting. Any combination of these signs and symptoms may be present.
The disease lasts a few days, recovery is complete and a diagnosis of poliomyelitis is rarely
made. The tendency is to refer to the above as
abortive polio. In 4 to 8 percent of the cases
the disease is slightly more severe, and in addition to the above there are indications of CNS
involvement. The patient presents with stiffness
and pain in the back and neck. There are indications of meningeal irritation and a high spinal
fluid cell count. The disease subsides in 2 to
5 days and recovery is complete. This is often
referred to as nonparalytic polio. In about
1 percent or less of the cases, several days
following the above minor illness, the signs and
symptoms reappear and progress to flaccid paralysis. The paralytic phase may occur without, or

as a continuation of, the minor illness. In
classic cases of paralytic polio the disease is
biphasic. The onset of paralysis is abrupt and
reaches its maximum following the fifth day of
its appearance.

    2. *Pathogenesis*. The virus enters by the
oral route by ingestion and multiplies in the
oropharyngeal and intestinal mucosa. It is subsequently absorbed by the lymphatic system from
where it enters the blood stream and is spread
to other susceptible tissues such as viscera and
brown fat. It is the multiplication in these
tissues that is responsible for the persistent
viremia. The virus may next reach the CNS either
by spread along the axons of the peripheral
nerves or by passing the blood brain barrier.
The primary route is probably the latter. The
virus multiplies in neurons, with anterior horn
cells of the spinal cord being most often involved. Lesions may also be seen in the medulla
and brain stem and motor cortex. The distribution of lesions parallels the severity and type
of clinical response.

    3. *Pathology*. The lesions of poliovirus are
present mainly in the nervous system, and are
found wherever neurons have been destroyed. Lymphocytes, plasma cells and macrophages collect
around the affected neurons. There is a perivascular inflammation (perivascular cuffing) of
lymphocytes around arterioles and venules. The
lesions are most often seen in the anterior horns
and to a lesser extent in the autonomic and sensory column of the spinal cord. Neurons may be
attacked but not destroyed and undergo a reversibl
chromatolysis of the Nissl bodies. The brain
lesions involve the motor cells of the reticular
substance of the medulla and pons, the vestibular
nuclei and related centers. The cerebral cortex
lesions are limited to motor and pre-motor areas.
The visual and auditory areas are not involved.
Edema and congestion may be found in liver, spleen
and other viscera.

    4. *Immune Response*. Antibody response is
specific and is permanent to the type causing
the infection. There is some cross-reactivity
among the polioviruses which may be demonstrated
by neutralization, between types 1 and 2, a

slight amount between types 2 and 3, but none
between 1 and 3.   There is a moderate heterotypic
antibody response following infection with a
second type poliovirus, especially types 1 and 2.
The degree of cross-protection conferred by this
response is not well defined.   Complement fixing
antibodies first appear at about the eighth day
following exposure, peak at 8 weeks and persist
for about 2 years.   Neutralizing antibodies appear at about 6 days, peak at 2 to 6 weeks and
remain in low concentration for the life of the
invididual.

    5.   *Prognosis*.   Less than 1 percent of the
cases of poliomyelitis proceed as far as the
paralytic stage.   Eighty to 90 percent of these
cases show permanent flaccid paralysis of the
legs alone or leg involvement in association
with that of the trunk, arms, etc.   Paralysis of
the arms alone occurs in less than 10 percent of
the cases.   If the nuclei in the cervical and
dorsal spinal column are attacked, paralysis of
the respiratory muscles ensues and is often fatal.
Paralysis reaches a maximum within a few days
after onset and often some degree of recovery
follows.   The overall mortality following the
paralytic stage is about 10 percent.   There are
no known congenital effects due to poliomyelitis
during pregnancy.

C.   DIAGNOSIS.
    1.   *Clinical*.   The diagnosis is not difficult
during epidemics or when the disease reaches the
paralytic stage.   A febrile episode, usually biphasic, followed by flaccid paralysis is characteristic of polio.   Abortive and nonparalytic
cases are impossible to diagnose clinically.
Cerebrospinal fluid values are useful; in polio
the sugar is normal, the protein slightly elevated,
and there are increased leucocytes (10 to 400 per
cubic mm).
    2.   *Laboratory*.
      a.   Virus Isolation. The virus is present
in the throat a few days after onset of the clinical signs and symptoms.   It persists in the

throat for a period of 10 to 14 days and in the
feces for from 5 to 14 weeks. Specimens taken
from these sources are treated with antibiotics
and fungistatic agents and inoculated into human
or monkey kidney tissue cultures. In the event
the specimen cannot be sent directly to the laboratory it should be stored frozen until used.
The virus is rarely isolated from spinal fluid.
The inoculated cells are examined daily for the
development of enterovirus cytopathogenicity.
The isolate is then identified by neutralization
with specific poliovirus type 1, 2 or 3 antiserum.
The minimum elapsed time for isolation and identification is about one week. Poliovirus isolated
from throat or stool must be characterized as
either "wild" or vaccine strain. This is based
on the ability of the "wild" strain only to grow
at $40^{\circ}C$.

      b. <u>Serology</u>. Complement fixation tests
using acute serum collected early in the infection and convalescent serum collected 10 to 14
days later serve as a method of serologic diagnosis. Neutralization tests may also be used.
In either case a fourfold increase in antibody
titer is considered diagnostic, in the absence
of recent poliovirus vaccination.

D. TREATMENT. There is no specific chemotherapy
for poliovirus. The treatment is supportive and,
depending upon the type of anatomical response,
may involve tracheotomy or use of a respirator.

E. EPIDEMIOLOGY. Poliovirus is detectable and
persists for several weeks in the stools of 95
to 100 percent of infected persons. This accounts for the main method of spread of the virus,
the fecal-oral route. Contamination of food and
water supplies with poliovirus-carrying sewage is
possible, but epidemics traceable to these sources
have not been proven. The role of insects and
shellfish in polio transmission is also not clear.
It is possible that the virus might also be
spread by the respiratory route, since it is known
that it is present in the oropharyngeal mucus.

The disease is endemic throughout the year in
tropical countries, and in temperate climates
occurs mainly in summer and early fall. The major incidence is in the 6-month to 9-year age
groups. The disease is rarely seen in the 0-6-
month age group owing to the presence of maternal
antibody. It is also rare in the over-20-year-
old age group owing to active natural immunity
acquired at an earlier age. In the years just
prior to the use of artificial immunization
against polio there was a shift in incidence to
the early teenage years. It must be remembered
that over 90 percent of the infections are nonparalytic and most never come to the attention
of a physician. Man is the only known reservoir
of the virus. This disease is now rarely seen
owing to the widespread use of poliovirus vaccination.

F.   PREVENTION.
     1. _Passive Immunization_. Pooled human gamma
globulin can provide protection against the paralytic effects of poliovirus for about 3 weeks.
It is most effective when given before exposure
or early in the incubation period. Its use is
based on the knowledge that most of the population has antibodies to poliovirus, and pooling
and concentrating enough serum specimens should
provide protection against all three polio types.
It is administered intramuscularly 0.15 ml per
pound of body weight.
     2. _Active Immunization_.
         a.   Inactivated Polio Vaccine (IPV).
This vaccine consists of an aqueous suspension
of formaldehyde-inactivated polioviruses type 1,
2 and 3. It is prepared in rhesus monkey kidney
cells grown _in vitro_, and is given as three
intramuscular or subcutaneous inoculations 4 to
6 weeks apart. A booster inoculation is given
every 2 to 3 years. After a primary series of
three doses, the antibody conversion rate is 92
to 100 percent for all three types. Antibody
produced prevents invasion of the CNS and paralysis by neutralizing any poliovirus which enters

the blood stream. It does not inhibit multiplication of the virus in the alimentary tract and
thus carriage and dissemination of the virus may
follow contact with polio cases. It does, however, prevent infection of the oropharyngeal
mucosa and therefore would prevent the suspected
respiratory transmission route.

        b. <u>Live Attenuated Polio Virus Vaccines</u>.
            1) General properties--the oral
polio vaccines consist of live virus which has
lost its neurovirulence owing to attenuation by
passage in tissue culture. The lack of neurovirulence is demonstrated by intramuscular and
intracranial inoculation into monkeys. The vaccine is prepared in tissue cultures of primary
rhesus monkey kidney cells. A stable line of
passaged human embryonic lung (WI-38) cells was
licensed in 1972 for vaccine production. The
advantages of passaged cells over primary cells
lies in the safety checking that can be done on
the passaged cells prior to use. Primary cultures
require that for every lot of vaccine produced,
new animals must be killed to provide tissue.
Since monkeys are known to harbor latent viruses,
this presents a definite problem in safety checking. The WI-38 cells have been used for vaccine
production in Canada for some years without any
problem.

           The live attenuated vaccines are
given by the oral route in a dose of about 10^5
tissue culture infectious particles for each
type of virus. This is sufficient to infect the
gastrointestinal tract and results in multiplication and excretion of virus for a period of 4 to
6 weeks and occasionally as long as 3 months.
Virus is first excreted at about 24 hours and
reaches a peak concentration of 10^4 to 10^6 particles per gram of feces at 1 to 2 weeks. Antibody conversion results in 90 to 100 percent of
the recipients. The immunity produced, unlike
that produced by inactivated polio vaccine, prevents reinfection of the gastrointestinal tract
by natural "wild" type virus. Thus, with the
live virus vaccine, it should be possible to

eradicate polio from society. The safety record
of the vaccines is excellent. The paralysis
rate is 0.06 per million doses in recipients
and 0.14 per million doses in contacts of vaccinees. The higher rate in contacts may be due
to prevailing contraindications to the use of the
vaccine for these persons.

      2) Monovalent oral polio vaccine--
the monovalent vaccine consists of separate
aqueous suspensions of poliovirus types 1, 2 and
3. The first dose is recommended at 6 to 12
weeks of age and the second and third at 6 to 8
week intervals. The sequence is type 2 first,
type 1 second, and type 3 third. Children and
adolescents may be vaccinated using the same
schedule. Routine immunization of adults in the
continental United States is not desirable unless
there is special risk or in epidemics. A single
booster dose of trivalent vaccine is recommended
upon entering kindergarten or first grade. Children who have not been vaccinated at that time
should be given a complete primary series.

      3) Trivalent oral polio vaccine--
the trivalent vaccine is a single aqueous suspension of all three poliovirus types. The first
dose is recommended at 6 to 12 weeks of age, the
second 6 to 8 weeks later, and a third dose 8 to
12 months following the second dose. A booster
dose of trivalent vaccine is recommended upon
entering kindergarten or first grade. Children
and adolescents may be vaccinated using the same
primary vaccination schedule.

      4) Contraindications--the live vac-
cines should not be given in cases of leukemia,
lymphoma, general malignancy or when resistance
is lowered by therapy with antimetabolites, radiation, steroids or alkylating agents. Pregnancy
is *not* a contraindication to use.

G. CONTROL. The spread of the disease cannot be
controlled by quarantine of patients or contacts
since a large number of infections are subclinical.
Proper precautions should be observed in the handling of fecal and oral discharges from hospitalized cases.

Chapter XXVI

RHINOVIRUSES (COMMON COLD)

A. PROPERTIES OF THE VIRUSES. Rhinoviruses contain RNA as their genetic material, are 15 to 30
nm in size, have cubic icosahedral symmetry, do
not have an envelope and are classified as members of the picornavirus group. Over 100 antigenic types have been shown to exist. There is
no common group antigen and type identification
is carried out by neutralization in tissue culture. They are resistant to ether and chloroform
but are inactivated by boiling, 56°C for 30 minutes and 1 percent formaldehyde. Unlike the
enterovirus subgroup, the rhinoviruses are sensitive to acid (pH 3-5). Infectivity is retained
for weeks at refrigerator temperature (4°C) and
for years at -70°C or lower.

B. HOST RESPONSE TO INFECTION.
    1. *Incubation Period, Signs and Symptoms*.
The incubation period is 1 to 5 days and the onset is insidious with sneezing, chills, headache,
nasal discharge and occasionally low-grade fever.
The disease usually runs its course in 4 to 10
days, with a moderation of signs and symptoms
after the first few days. It is not uncommon to
have 1 to 3 attacks during the winter season.
    2. *Pathogenesis*. The virus enters by way
of the upper respiratory tract and multiplies
in the nasal mucosa and pharynx. It appears to
be confined to growth in these tissues and is
present in nasal secretions from a few days before
until 2 to 7 days after onset of symptoms. As
far as is known the viruses are not present in
other body secretions.
    3. *Pathology*. There is no distinctive
pathology.
    4. *Immune Response*. The most important im-
munoglobulin in immunity to rhinoviruses is

specific IgA, especially that present in the nasal
secretions. Reinfection with a homotypic virus
appears to be unrelated to the level of serum IgG.
It is also possible to demonstrate resistance to
heterotypic rhinoviruses for several weeks following infection with any type and to homotypic virus
for several years. It is possible that the short-
term heterotypic resistance is due to interferon.
    5. _Prognosis_. The common cold is an ir-
ritating and economically costly disease, but
little else. Occasionally there have been complications associated with chronic bronchitis or
bronchopneumonia, but the disease is normally
self-resolving with complete recovery.

C. DIAGNOSIS.
    1. _Clinical_. Owing to the mild nature of the
disease, a clinical diagnosis is rarely required.
The signs and symptoms are characteristic enough,
and recur often enough, so that lay persons become
their own diagnosticians.
    2. _Laboratory_.
        a. Isolation of the Virus. Rhinoviruses
may be isolated in primary cultures of human embryonic or rhesus monkey kidney or diploid human
lung cells. The rhinoviruses may be divided into
two broad groups on the basis of their ability to
grow in either human cell cultures only (H viruses)
or in both human and monkey cultures (M viruses).
In humans the antibody response to M viruses is
greater than that to H viruses. Isolation is carried out at 33°C in cultures rotated in "roller
drums" at about 1 revolution per minute. They
produce an "enterovirus-like" CPE. The specimens
of choice are nose and throat swabs or washings
collected anytime from onset of symptoms until
2 to 5 days later. Neutralization with specific
type antiserum is the only method for exact identification. As might be expected, isolation
studies are rarely done except as a part of
epidemiologic or other research studies.
        b. Serology. Acute and convalescent studies
are seldom done, and are not requested as a routine
laboratory practice. Type-specific serum-neutral-
izing antibodies can be demonstrated 14 to 21 days

following infection. Complement fixation tests
are less specific and seldom used.

D. TREATMENT. There is no specific treatment.

E. EPIDEMIOLOGY. Rhinoviruses are worldwide in
distribution and there is a greater incidence of
infections in children and young adults than in
older age groups. The largest number of cases
occur in late fall, winter and early spring.
The transmission is person to person by way of
the respiratory tract.

F. PREVENTION.
    1. _Active Immunization_. There are no vac-
cines available and none in prospect.
    2. _Passive Immunization_. Passive protection
is not practiced with rhinoviruses.
    3. _Vitamin C Prophylaxis_. Several studies
have been conducted in humans to determine whether
or not vitamin C has any effect in preventing the
common cold. The results have been conflicting;
some studies showed fewer colds in the vitamin
group, others could find no difference between
treated and placebo groups. It is not possible
to make a decision regarding its usefulness at
this time.

G. CONTROL. There are no specific control
measures.

Chapter XXVII

REOVIRUSES (1, 2, 3)

A. PROPERTIES OF THE VIRUS. Reoviruses (Respiratory Enteric Orphan viruses) contain double-stranded RNA as their genetic material, are about 60 to 80 nm in size, have a cubic icosahedral symmetry, do not have an envelope and possess a hemagglutinin for human type O red blood cells. Three antigenic types have been demonstrated by neutralization or hemagglutination inhibition. There is also a common complement fixing antigen. Reoviruses are classified as members of the diplornavirus (reovirus) group. They are resistant to ether and chloroform but are inactivated by formalin, drying, and 56°C for 45 minutes. They retain their infectivity for years when stored at -70°C.

B. HOST RESPONSE TO INFECTION.
   1. _Incubation Period, Signs and Symptoms_. Despite the fact that reoviruses have been shown to commonly infect man and most animals, no disease has as yet been directly attributed to them. They have occasionally been isolated from the throat and stools of cases of respiratory disease or diarrhea, but their role in these diseases is not clear. Adult volunteers inoculated intranasally with reoviruses failed to develop any clear-cut signs or symptoms. The presence of reovirus antibodies in the adult human population (60 to 80 percent by age 20) attests to their prevalence.
   2. _Pathogenesis_. Little is known about the pathogenesis of reovirus infections. The virus probably enters by way of the oral cavity or respiratory tract and multiplies in the respiratory tissue and intestine. The nature and extent of the viremia if it occurs are not known.

   3. *Pathology*. No distinctive pathology has
been associated with reovirus infections.
   4. *Immune Response*. It has been shown by
means of human volunteer studies that hemagglutination inhibiting, complement fixing and neutralizing antibodies appear in about 10 days and peak
about 2 to 3 weeks following inoculation. They
remain at a high level for several months before
gradually declining. Antibodies are present
thereafter for years, perhaps for life, but
whether this is due to a booster effect from reinfection or to persistence of antibody *per se* is
not known.
   5. *Prognosis*. Human diseases in which reoviruses are the suspected but not proven etiological agents are mild respiratory syndromes
and gastroenteritis. In either case the disease
is self-resolving with no complications.

C. DIAGNOSIS.
   1. *Clinical*. No characteristic clinical
picture.
   2. *Laboratory*.
      a. Isolation of the Virus. Isolation is
most frequently accomplished by inoculation of
cell cultures of rhesus monkey kidney or human
embryonic lung or kidney, or HeLa cells with
throat or rectal swabs or stool samples. These
specimens should be collected as soon as possible
after the onset of disease, and if not used within a few hours of collection, they should be
stored frozen. Reoviruses produce a nonspecific
granular type degeneration in inoculated cultures.
Characteristic cytoplasmic inclusions are readily
seen in stained preparations. Viral identification is usually accomplished by hemagglutination-
inhibition.
      b. Serology. Complement fixing (CF),
hemagglutination inhibiting (HI) and neutralizing antibodies appear by 10 to 14 days and peak
at 3 weeks. The CF antibodies are group-specific
while the HI antibodies are more type-specific.
There are heterotypic HI antibodies produced to
reovirus types 2 and 3 following infection with

type 1. The determination of neutralizing antibodies is the only serological method that is
type-specific. However, the HI test is most
commonly used because of its ease of performance
and greater sensitivity. Serum should be collected early after disease onset and at 2 to 3
weeks. A fourfold or greater increase in titer
is considered diagnostic.

D. TREATMENT. There is no specific treatment.

E. EPIDEMIOLOGY. The reoviruses are undoubtedly
transmitted by the fecal-oral or respiratory route.
It has been shown by experimental inoculation of
human volunteers that the virus is present in the
stools and respiratory tract for up to 10 days
following administration. Studies have also
shown that reoviruses may be isolated with the
greatest frequency from humans under natural circumstances in late summer, fall and early winter.
Reovirus infections are found throughout the
world in man as well as monkeys, rodents, cattle
and other mammals.

F. PREVENTION. No preventive measures are available.

G. CONTROL. There are no specific control measures.

Chapter XXVIII

RABIES

A. PROPERTIES OF THE VIRUS. Rabies virus contains RNA as its genetic material, has a helical symmetry, possesses an envelope and is bullet-shaped with dimensions of 70 by 175 nm. It is classified as a member of the Rhabdovirus group. posseses a hemagglutinin for goose erythrocytes and has only one known antigenic type. Rabies virus is rapidly destroyed by sunlight, ultra-violet radiation, boiling or temperatures of 54 to 56°C for one hour. It is inactivated by ether, chloroform, formalin, and strong acids and bases. It is resistant to phenol, alcohol, and merthiolate. It may be preserved in the active state for years by freezing at -70°C.

B. HOST RESPONSE TO VIRUS INFECTION.
   1. _Incubation Period, Signs and Symptoms_.
The incubation period of rabies averages from 30 to 90 days, with a range of 2 weeks to 5 months. There have been certain rare instances when it has been as short as 10 days or as long as 8 months. The prodromal symptoms, which last for a period of 2 to 4 days, are headache, malaise, low-grade temperature and nervousness. Quite early in the disease there is usually a tingling at the site of the animal bite. This occurs in about 80 percent of the cases and favors a diagnosis of rabies. Signs include muscle tics, overactive facial expression, rapid pulse rate and increased muscle tone. One of the outstanding characteristics of rabies is hydrophobia, or fear of water. This arises due to the reflex irritability of the throat muscles related to the act of swallowing. Fluid, which comes into contact with the fauces, produces painful spasmodic contractions of these muscles and accessory muscles of respiration. As the disease progresses there are increased excitation and convulsive seizures interspersed

with periods of quiescence. Usually the patient
dies during an acute excitement phase during a
convulsion. In certain cases, where the excitement phase is survived, the patient becomes quiet
and there are generalized paralysis, apathy, stupor,
coma and death. Persons developing rabies following a dog bite often die within ten days.

  2. *Pathogenesis*. The virus travels from the
site of the animal bite along the nerve trunk
pathways in a centripetal direction to the central
nervous system. The spinal cord and brain become
infected and the spread of the virus is then cen-
trifugal by way of the nerve trunk routes. It is
in this manner that the virus is spread to the
salivary gland. The virus multiplies only in
nerve cells and a viremia has not been demonstrated.

  3. *Pathology*. Postmortem examination does
not show any gross pathological lesions. The
meninges appear normal and the cerebrospinal fluid
findings are normal. Histological examination
shows nonspecific lesions similar to those seen
in fatal cases of viral encephalitis. The changes
observed are petechial hemorrhage around blood
vessels, perivascular lymphocytic cuffing and
gliosis. The neurons show pyknosis of the nucleus
and ballooning of the cytoplasm. This nerve cell
destruction is extensive in the cerebral and cere-
bellar cortices, pons, medulla and thalamus. The
medulla most often presents the maximum pathologic
alteration. The spinal cord shows hyperemia and
perivascular infiltration. There is extensive
neuronal destruction in the posterior horns. The
lesion characteristic of rabies is the *Negri body*.
These inclusions are most abundant in Ammon's
horn of the hippocampus, the pyramidal cell layer
of the cerebral cortex, the Purkinje cell layer
of the cerebellum and in large neurons of the
basal ganglia. They are found in the cytoplasm
of neurons and are 2 to 10 microns in size and
oval or round in shape. When the tissue is prepared with Seller's or a similar stain, the Negri
bodies appear acidophilic with internal basophilic granules.

4. *Immune Response*. Following infection or vaccination, complement fixing, hemagglutination inhibiting and virus neutralizing antibodies are produced. Neutralizing antibody persists for a number of years and Nt is the serological test of choice for demonstrating the immune response. In addition to the antibodies listed above there is a virus-specific antibody present which lyses infected cells in the presence of complement. It is possible that this antibody might play a role in the pathogenesis of the disease.

5. *Prognosis*. It has always been considered, and well substantiated, that once clinical signs and symptoms of rabies develop in a human the disease is invariably fatal. A few poorly documented cases had been reported prior to 1970, but it was not until this time that a well-substantiated human rabies recovery was reported. The case involved a 6-year-old boy who was bitten on the thumb by a bat which was later proven to be rabid. The child developed clinical rabies 20 days after exposure and 2 days following a 14-day course of duck embryo rabies vaccine. Rabies serum neutralization titers reached a level of 1:63,000 at 3 months and the child had completely recovered by 6 months after onset. It is probable that the treatment to prevent hypoxia, intracranial hypertension, cardiac arrhythmia, superinfection and seizures contributed materially to the child's recovery. At the very least, the classic textbook statement that human clinical rabies is 100 percent fatal will become obsolete, and physicians confronted with a rabies victim will treat the patient with hope and not hopelessness.

C. DIAGNOSIS.

1. *Clinical*. Rabies and its association with an animal bite is well known throughout the world. It is for this reason that in suspected rabies cases information concerning a fairly recent animal bite will be given by the patient himself. In lieu of this information, the classical signs and symptoms together with a scarred-

over animal bite are useful in establishing a
diagnosis. In many cases, the patient will have
consulted a physician within a short period of
time following exposure and may have been sub-
jected to anti-rabies treatment. There may be
occasions when a differential diagnosis has to
be established between rabies, tetanus and post-
rabies vaccine encephalitis. Tetanus from
Clostridium tetani contamination at the site of
the bite will usually have a much shorter incubation time than rabies. Post-rabies vaccine
encephalitis which is quite rare occurs most
often after the 7th rabies Semple (rabbit brain)
type vaccine inoculation in persons who have had
previous exposure to the vaccine.

   2. *Laboratory*.

     a. <u>Isolation of the Virus</u>. The finding
of Negri bodies in brain tissue of humans is
pathognomonic of rabies. When they cannot be
found it is necessary to resort to animal inoculation. The specimens of choice from brain tissue are cerebral cortex, medulla and basal ganglia. The material is ground in a mortar and
pestle, diluted and inoculated intracerebrally
into albino mice. If the specimen is positive,
convulsions or paralysis will be seen within 6 to
10 days. Rabies is then confirmed by demonstrating Negri bodies in brain tissue of these mice.
Saliva, collected from under the tongue, and cerebrospinal fluid may also be used for rabies virus
isolation.

     b. <u>Fluorescent Antibody (FA) Tests</u>.
Rapid confirmation of suspected rabies in animals
may be obtained by using the direct fluorescent
rabies antibody (FRA) test on smears of brain,
cornea or salivary gland. The smears are over-
layed with fluorescein isothiocyanate labeled
rabies hyperimmune serum and viewed with a fluorescent microscope. This test is usually carried out concurrently with smears stained with
Seller's stain and examined for the presence of
Negri bodies. The results of these tests are
usually available within 24 hours. The same
techniques may be applied to human postmortem

specimens.

      c.   Serology. Specific antibody against
rabies may be detected by virus neutralization
in mice or serum indirect FA titration. A rapid
fluorescent focus inhibition test (RFFIT) is
finding greater application for measuring levels
of rabies virus Nt antibody. In this test, dilu-
tions of patient's serum are reacted with a standard dose of a "fixed" or attenuated strain of
rabies virus. Virus neutralization is indicated
by a reduction of invasive foci in inoculated
cell cultures when reacted with a fluorescent
anti-rabies conjugate. The tests may be used to
confirm a diagnosis or to detect the level of
antibody produced in response to vaccination.

      d.   Negri Bodies. These inclusions are
discussed under Pathology.

D.   TREATMENT. There is no specific therapy for
rabies once the clinical disease develops. The
aggressive treatment used in the one documented
human rabies recovery probably contributed to
its favorable outcome. It is discussed under
Prognosis. Treatment following suspected or
known exposure is covered under Prevention.

E.   EPIDEMIOLOGY. Rabies is principally a disease of carnivorous biting animals such as dogs,
cats, foxes, skunks, and wolves. In the
United States in 1971 there were a total of
4310 cases of animal rabies reported. Of the
total, 2018 were in skunks, 671 in foxes, 465
in bats, 390 in cattle, 230 in dogs, 190 in
raccoons, and 336 in miscellaneous wild and
domestic animals. The high incidence in bats
presents an interesting problem since they may
have a healthy carrier rate as high as 1 percent. The reservoir of infection is in the
above wild animals, and man or his domestic
animals are "chance" hosts. The risk of acquiring rabies from rats, mice, squirrels or guinea
pigs is quite low.

      Infection depends upon the entrance of virus-
laden saliva into a wound caused by the bite of

a rabid animal. Virus is present in the saliva
of the animal from the onset of clinical signs
until death. It is found in saliva of from 50
to 90 percent of infected animals and has a
slightly higher prevalence in skunks and foxes
than in dogs. It is possible to transmit the
disease by introducing the virus into cuts or
abrasions while "playing" with an infected
animal. Recent reports indicate that under
certain highly specialized circumstances aerosol
transmission by bats is possible.

Although there are only about 1000 cases of
human rabies reported annually worldwide, there
are nearly a million human post-exposure rabies
immunizations. The average annual rate over the
past ten years in man in the United States has
been two cases per year. Rabies is worldwide in
distribution and has no particular seasonal incidence.

F.   PREVENTION.
    1. *Animals*.
        a.   Live Attenuated Rabies Virus Vaccines
for Use in Animals. There are five licensed live
attenuated rabies virus vaccines for use in
animals. They are prepared in chick embryo,
canine kidney, or porcine kidney tissue cultures.
In dogs the first dose is given at 3 to 4 months
and the second at one year of age. The duration
of immunity is 3 years and a booster shot is
given at that time. The inoculations are given
intramuscularly and may be either a low egg passage (LEP) or high egg passage (HEP) type vaccine. The LEP vaccines should not be used in
animals other than dogs. In cats or cattle, high
egg passage or porcine kidney vaccines are recommended. The schedule of immunizations is slightly
different for individual vaccines, and manufacturer's directions should be followed.
        b.   Inactivated Rabies Vaccines for Use
in Animals. There are five licensed inactivated
rabies vaccines for use in animals. They are
prepared in hamster kidney or caprine nervous
tissue cell cultures. These vaccines are given

as two doses 3 to 4 weeks apart with the first
inoculation given at 3 to 4 months of age. A
booster dose is given annually and the duration
of immunity is one year.
     2. _Humans_. The "Recommendations of the
Public Health Service Advisory Committee on
Immunization Practices: Rabies Prophylaxis"
are reproduced below in their entirety.*

G.   RABIES PROPHYLAXIS.
     1. _Introduction_. Although human rabies is
rare in the United States, thousands of persons
receive rabies prophylaxis each year. Management of those who possibly have been exposed to
rabies infection is of paramount importance.
The following is a current interpretation of both
the risk of infection and the efficacy of treatment. It incorporates many basic concepts of
the World Health Organization Expert Committee
on Rabies.
     The problem of whether or not to immunize
those bitten, scratched, or otherwise exposed
to rabies by animals suspected of being infectious is a perplexing one for physicians. All
available methods of systemic treatment are
complicated by instances of adverse reactions,
a few of which have resulted in death or permanent disability. Furthermore, decisions on
management must be made immediately, because the
longer treatment is postponed, the less likely
it is to be effective.
     Data on the efficacy of active and passive
immunization after rabies exposure have come
principally from studies in animals. Because
rabies has occasionally developed in humans who
had received anti-rabies prophylaxis, the data
have been questioned. Evidence from laboratory

---

*Morbidity and Mortality World Reports: Volume 16,
 No. 19, 1967; revised Volume 18, No. 43-Supple-
 ment 1969; revised Volume 21, No. 25-Supplement 1972.

and field experience in many areas of the world,
however, indicates that post-exposure prophylaxis
is usually effective when appropriately used.

  a. <u>Rabies in the United States</u>. Rabies
in humans has decreased from an average of
22 cases per year in 1946 to 1950 to only 1 or
2 cases per year since 1963. Rabies in domestic
animals has diminished similarly. In 1946, for
example, there were more than 8000 cases of
rabies in dogs, compared with 230 in 1971. Thus,
the likelihood of humans being exposed to rabies
by domestic animals has decreased greatly
although bites by dogs and cats continue to be
responsible for the overwhelming majority of
anti-rabies treatment.

  In contrast, the disease in wildlife--espe-
cially skunks, foxes, raccoons, and bats--has
become increasingly prominent in recent years,
accounting for more than 70 percent of all reported cases of animal rabies in 1971. Wild
animals constitute the most important source of
infection for man and domestic animals in the
United States today. In 1971, only a single
state reported no wildlife rabies.

  b. <u>Anti-rabies Treatment in the
United States</u>. More than 30,000 persons receive
post-exposure anti-rabies treatment each year.
However, there is no information on the number
of persons actually exposed to rabid animals.

  In the United States, nervous tissue origin
rabies vaccine of the Semple type (NTV) was
used almost exclusively until 1957, when duck
embryo origin vaccine (DEV) was licensed. More
than 90 percent of those who received rabies
prophylaxis in the United States in 1971 were
given DEV.

  2. *Rabies Vaccines*.

  a. <u>Duck Embryo Vaccine (DEV)</u>. Prepared
from embryonated duck eggs infected with a fixed
virus and inactivated with betapropiolactone.

  b. <u>Nervous Tissue Vaccine (NTV)</u>. Prepared from rabbit brain infected with a fixed
virus and inactivated with phenol (Semple type)
or inactivated with ultraviolet irradiation.

    c.   <u>Antigenicity of Vaccines</u>. The anti-
genicity of NTV is often higher than that of DEV
when tested in experimental animals. However,
all lots of both vaccines must pass minimum
potency tests established by the Division of
Biologics Standards.* There is evidence that
the serum antibody response in humans is detectable sooner with DEV, but the eventual level of
response is frequently higher with NTV.

    d.   <u>Effectiveness of Vaccines in Humans</u>.
In the United States, comparative effectiveness
of vaccines can be judged only by reported fail-
ures. During the years 1957 through 1971 when
both vaccines were available, there were 6 rabies
deaths among the 125,000 NTV-treated persons
(1:20,800) and 12 among the 310,000 treated with
DEV (1:25,800).

    e.   Reactions. Erythema, pruritus, pain,
and tenderness at the site of inoculation are
common with both DEV and NTV. Systemic responses,
including low-grade fever or rarely shock, may
occasionally occur late in the course of therapy
with either vaccine, usually after 5 to 8 doses.
In rare instances, serious reactions have occurred
after the first dose of DEV or NTV, particularly
in persons previously sensitized with vaccines
containing avian or rabbit brain tissue.

    Neuroparalytic reactions occur rarely with
DEV. They much more frequently follow NTV, especially after repeated courses of treatment
with this preparation.

    f.   <u>Choice of Vaccine</u>. Treatment-failure
rates for the two vaccines are not significantly
different; therefore, the lower incidence of
central nervous system reactions with DEV makes
it preferable to NTV.

    3.   *Rationale of Treatment*. Every exposure
to possible rabies infection must be individually
evaluated.

---

*Now the Bureau of Biologics, Food and Drug
  Administration.

In the United States, the following factors
should be considered before specific anti-rabies
treatment is initiated:

Species of Biting Animal. Carnivorous
animals (especially skunks, foxes, coyotes, raccoons, dogs and cats) and bats are more likely
to be infective than other animals. Bites of
rabbits, squirrels, chipmunks, rats, and mice,
seldom, if ever, call for rabies prophylaxis.

Circumstances of Biting Incident. An
UNPROVOKED attack is more likely to mean that
the animal is rabid. (Bites during attempts to
feed or handle an apparently healthy animal
should generally be regarded as PROVOKED.)

Type of Exposure. Rabies is transmitted by
inoculation of infectious saliva through the
skin. Thus, the likelihood that rabies infection will result from exposure to a rabid animal
varies with the nature and extent of the exposure.
Two categories of exposure should be considered:

> Bite wounds--any penetration of the
> skin by teeth.
> Non-bite wounds--scratches, abrasions,
> or open wounds.

Vaccination Status of Biting Animal. A prop-
erly immunized animal has only a minimal chance
of developing rabies and transmitting the virus.

Presence of Rabies in Region. If adequate
laboratory and field records indicate that there
is no rabies infection in a domestic species
within a given region, local health officials
are justified in considering this in recommendations on anti-rabies treatment following a bite
by the particular species.

4. *Management of Biting Animals.* A
healthy domestic dog or cat that bites a person
should be captured, confined, and observed by
a veterinarian for 10 days. (The commonly used
5 to 7 day observation period may not always be
adequate.) Any illness in the animal should be
reported immediately to the local health department.

If the dog or cat develops signs suggestive
of rabies, the animal should be sacrificed and

the head removed and shipped under refrigeration
to a qualified laboratory designated by the
local or State Health Department for examination.

Early signs of rabies in wild or stray
animals cannot be interpreted reliably; therefore,
any such animal that bites or scratches a person
should be killed at once (without unnecessary
damage to the head) and the brain examined for
evidence of rabies.

If examination of the brain by fluorescent
antibody technique is negative for rabies, the
bitten person need not be treated.

5. *Local Treatment of Wounds*. *Immediate
and thorough local treatment of all bite wounds
and scratches is perhaps the most effective means
of preventing rabies*. Experimentally, the incidence of rabies in animals can be markedly reduced
by local therapy alone.

a. First-aid Treatment to be Carried
Out Immediately. Copious flushing with soap and
water.

b. Treatment by or Under Direction of
Physician.

1) Thorough flushing and cleansing
into the wound with soap solution. Quaternary
ammonium compounds may also be used.*

2) If anti-rabies serum is indicated
(see Passive Immunization), up to one-half of
the total dose should be thoroughly infiltrated
around the wound. As in all instances when horse
serum is to be used, a careful history should be
taken and tests for hypersensitivity performed.

3) Tetanus prophylaxis and measures
to control bacterial infection, as indicated.

6. *Post-exposure Prophylaxis*. The following recommendations are intended only as a guide.
They may be modified according to knowledge of
the species of biting animal, circumstances surrounding the biting incident, vaccination status
of the animal, and presence of rabies in the
region.

---

*Such as Zephiran (benzyl ammonium chloride).
 All traces of soap should be removed before
 applying quaternary ammonium compounds, because
 soap neutralizes their activity.

a.   Active Immunization.
1)   Vaccine without serum--14 daily
injections of the vaccine in the dose recommended
by the manufacturer.
2)   Vaccine with serum--when serum
is used, 21 doses of vaccine are recommended.
These may be given as 21 daily doses or 14 doses
in the first 7 days (either as two separate injections or a double dose), and then 7 daily
doses. Two booster doses, the first 10 days and
the second at least 20 days after completion of
the primary course, are necessary to assure lasting protection.
3)   Precautions--vaccine should be
given subcutaneously in the abdomen, lower back,
or lateral aspect of thighs; rotation of sites is
recommended. Local reactions are common and do
not contraindicate continuing treatment.
When rabies vaccine must be given to a person
with a history of hypersensitivity, especially to
avian or rabbit tissues, antihistaminic drugs may
be given. Epinephrine is indicated in reactions
of the anaphylactoid type. If serious allergic
manifestations preclude continuation of prophylaxis with one vaccine, the other may be used.
If meningeal or neuroparalytic reactions
develop, vaccine treatment should be discontinued
altogether. Corticosteroids may interfere with
development of active immunity and should only
be used to treat neuroparalytic reactions.
b.   Passive Immunization. Hyperimmune
serum has proved effective in preventing rabies.
Its use in combination with vaccine is considered
the best post-exposure prophylaxis. However, the
only preparation of anti-rabies serum currently
available in the United States is of equine origin.*

---

*Human rabies immune globulin (HRIG) was licensed
 in July, 1974. It is prepared from human plasma
 pools with high rabies antibody titer obtained from
 rabies immunized volunteers. See Morbidity and
 Mortality Weekly Report: Volume 23, No. 33
 August 17, 1974.

Because horse serum has induced serum sickness
in at least 20 percent of those who have received
it, it should be used only when indicated.

Hyperimmune serum is recommended for ALL
BITES by animals in which rabies cannot be excluded and for non-bite exposure to animals
proved or suspected to be rabid (see accompanying guide). When indicated, anti-rabies serum
should be used regardless of the interval
between exposure and treatment.

The recommended dose of equine anti-rabies
serum is 40 IU/kg, *i.e.*, approximately 20 IU/lb
or 1000 IU (1 vial)/55 pounds. Up to 50 percent of the antiserum should be used to infiltrate the wound and the rest administered intramuscularly. As previously noted, when using
serum, a careful history must be obtained and
appropriate tests for hypersensitivity performed.

7. *Pre-exposure Prophylaxis*. The relatively
low frequence of reactions to DEV has made it
practical to offer pre-exposure immunization to
persons in high-risk groups: veterinarians,
animal handlers, certain laboratory workers, and
individuals, especially children, living in areas
of the world where rabies is a constant threat.
Others whose vocational or avocational pursuits
result in frequent contact with dogs, cats, foxes,
skunks, or bats should also be considered for
pre-exposure prophylaxis.

Two 1.0 ml injections of DEV given subcutaneously in the deltoid area 1 month apart should
be followed by a third dose 6 to 7 months after
the second dose. This series of three injections
can be expected to produce neutralizing antibody
in 80 to 90 percent of vaccinees by 1 month after
the third dose.

For more rapid immunization, three injections
of DEV, 1.0 ml each, should be given at weekly
intervals with a fourth dose 3 months later.
This schedule elicits an antibody response in
about 80 percent of the vaccinees.

All who receive the pre-exposure vaccination
should have serum tested for neutralizing antibody 3 to 4 weeks after the last injection.

Tests for rabies antibody can be arranged by state health department laboratories. If no antibody is detected, booster doses should be given until a response is demonstrated. Persons with continuing exposure should receive 1.0 ml boosters every 2 to 3 years.

When an immunized person with previously demonstrated rabies antibody is bitten by a rabid animal, it is suggested that he receive five daily doses of vaccine plus a booster dose 20 days later. Anti-rabies serum is not necessary in this case and, in fact, might inhibit a rapid anamnestic response. For non-bite exposures, an immunized person with antibody needs only a single dose of vaccine. If it is not known whether an exposed person ever had antibody, the complete post-exposure anti-rabies treatment should be given.

Post-Exposure Anti-Rabies Guide

The following recommendations are only a guide. They should be used in conjunction with knowledge of the animal species involved, circumstances of the bite or other exposure, vaccination status of the animal, and presence of rabies in the region.

Animal and its Condition		Treatment Kind of Exposure	
Species	Condition at Time of Attack	Bite*	Non-bite*
Wild: Skunk Fox Raccoon Bat	Regard as Rabid	S + V[1]	S + V[1]
Domestic: Dog	Healthy	None[2]	None[2]
	Escaped (unknown)	S + V[1]	V[3]
Cat	Rabid	S + V[1]	S + V[1]
Other	Consider individually--see "Rationale of Treatment"		

* see text definitions
V Rabies Vaccine
S Anti-rabies Serum
[1] Discontinue vaccine if fluorescent antibody (FA) tests of animal killed at time of attack are negative
[2] Begin S + V at first sign of rabies in biting dog or cat during holding period (10 days)
[3] 14 doses of DEV

    8. Accidental Inoculation with Live Rabies Virus Vaccine. Persons inadvertently inoculated with the Flury strain (attenuated rabies virus animal) vaccine are not considered at risk, and anti-rabies prophylaxis is not indicated. No information is available by which to judge risk from accidental inoculation of other attenuated strains in veterinary use.

Chapter XXIX

RUBELLA
(GERMAN MEASLES, 3-DAY MEASLES)

A. PROPERTIES OF THE VIRUS. Rubella virus contains RNA as its genetic material, is enveloped, is about 35 to 40 nm in size and has a cubic icosahedral symmetry. It is classified as an alphavirus in the togavirus group and possesses a hemagglutinin for one-day-old chicken as well as adult pigeon and duck red blood cells. There is only one known antigenic type. It is inactivated by ether, alcohol, drying, common disinfectants and weak solutions of phenol and formaldehyde. Its viability may be maintained for years by storage at -70°C.

B. HOST RESPONSE TO INFECTION.
    1. *Postnatal Rubella*.
        a. <u>Incubation Period, Signs and Symptoms</u>. The incubation period is usually 12 to 14 days but may be as short as 10 or as long as 21 days. Signs and symptoms are normally absent during the prodromal stage. Shortly before the appearance of the rash there may be a low-grade fever. The rash first appears on the face and head and spreads over the neck, trunk and extremities. It reaches full development within 24 hours and disappears at about 3 days. It consists of round, pink, slightly raised macules which are normally discrete but in some instances may become confluent. There is a lymphadenitis of the cervical and suboccipital nodes. The fever rarely exceeds 102°C and lasts for the duration of the rash (2 to 5 days).
        b. <u>Prognosis</u>. Postnatal rubella is a mild disease with little or no tendency toward secondary infections. Complications, when present, are usually seen as arthritis or arthralgia, especially in adult female patients. Rare complications are encephalitis and thrombocytopenic purpura.

c. Communicability. Rubella is less
contagious than measles and occurs in slightly
older age groups. The disease is normally spread
via the respiratory tract person to person by
direct contact. Infected persons are contagious
from one week before until a maximum of two weeks
after the rash. Carriers do not exist when the
infection is acquired postnatally, and immune
persons do not transmit the virus from an infected
to a nonimmune person.

d. Immune Response. In a primary infection the first antibodies detectable are the hemagglutination inhibiting (HI) and neutralizing
(Nt) antibodies which appear within 24 to 48 hours
after the rash. They peak 7 to 12 days later and
decline slowly over the years, but remain detectable in low titer for life. Complement fixing
antibody (CF) is detectable 4 days after onset
of rash, peaks at about 2 weeks and declines
rapidly so that it is no longer detectable 3 to
4 years post-infection. Primary infection results
in the production of rubella IgM followed in about
one week by IgG. Rubella HI and Nt antibody
remain throughout the life of the individual.
Upon reinfection, the secondary response results
exclusively in an increase of rubella IgG. Reinfection can occur, but nearly always results
in an inapparent infection.

e. Pathology. In uncomplicated rubella
there is no outstanding pathology. Aside from
the adenopathy of cervical, occipital, and posterior cervical nodes, there may be a slight
decrease in platelet count and discrete splenomegaly. In fatal post-infection encephalitis,
severe nonspecific neuronal degeneration with
slight perivascular infiltration and no demyelination has been reported.

2. *Congenital Effects*.

a. Congenital Syndrome Defined. In its
broadest terms this refers to any malformation
present at birth which occurred during fetal
development. This may be brought about by an
adverse effect during organogenesis or by

destruction of a formed organ. In virology, our
primary concern is with those defects caused by
viruses.

      b. <u>Congenital Rubella Syndrome</u>. Gregg,
in 1941, first noted an association between rubella infection in early pregnancy and cataracts
and low birth weight in neonates. Since his
observation, numerous studies by others, aided
by the isolation of rubella virus in 1962, have
expanded and clarified this relationship. The
reported risk of congenital rubella following
maternal infection varies considerably. However, a reasonable estimate based on several
studies of the probability of serious defects
correlated with gestation is: 0 to 4 weeks,
33 to 60 percent; 5 to 8 weeks, 25 to 33 percent; 9 to 12 weeks, 9 to 13 percent; 13 to 16
weeks, 2 to 5 percent. Infection after 16 weeks
gestation carries a slight but definite risk.
Overall, the risk in the first trimester is about
20 percent, with spontaneous abortions occurring
in about 10 to 15 percent of such pregnancies.

      c. <u>Pathogenesis</u>. In primary rubella,
viremia takes place from a week before until the
disappearance of the rash, and it is in this
period that placental infection could take place.
The infection is transient in placental tissue
but persists in the chorionic villi. Virus has
been recovered from placenta and membranes following abortion when rubella infection had taken
place during early pregnancy. The major effects
are seen when infection takes place during organogenesis (2 to 6 weeks following conception). The
virus may exert its effect by inhibiting mitosis
and/or producing chromosome breaks in developing organs. Malformations may also occur as a
result of cell necrosis caused by virus growth in
formed organs.

      d. <u>Congenital Rubella Syndrome, Clinical
Manifestations</u>. The effects on the fetus may be
seen in a wide variety of organs. In order of
frequency they are: intrauterine growth retardation (low birth weight, retarded growth), heart

(patent ductus arteriosus, septal defects, pulmonary stenosis), eye (cataracts, retinopathy,
microphthalmia, glaucoma), ear (deafness),
central nervous system (microcephaly, retarded
development), blood (thrombocytopenic purpura),
liver (hepatitis, jaundice, hepatosplenomegaly),
and bone (lesions, abnormal growth).

　　　e. Management. There is no specific
therapy for congenital rubella. The incidence
of virus excretion from the pharynges of these
babies has been reported as 84 percent shortly
after birth, dropping to 33 percent at 5 months
and 3 percent at 20 months. These infants can
spread the disease to susceptible persons and
obviously should be kept away from nonimmune
women in early pregnancy.

　　　f. Diagnosis. The only reliable diagnosis of congenital rubella is made using laboratory data and is based on any one of the following three criteria:

　　　1) Isolation of rubella virus from
the newborn.

　　　2) Demonstration of specific rubella
IgM in cord blood or serum obtained immediately
after birth.

　　　3) Persistence of detectable rubella
antibody in the infant in the absence of any
ensuing rubella infection, at 8 to 12 months.

Some explanation of points 2 and 3 is in
order. The fetus produces IgM in the second trimester but does not produce easily detectable
levels of IgG until after birth. If infected
in utero, rubella IgM produced *in utero* will be
present along with maternal rubella IgG (which
passes the placenta). Treatment of neonate
serum with 2-mercaptoethanol will disrupt the
IgM molecule, if present, but will not affect
IgG. Thus, a fourfold or greater decrease in
rubella HI antibody after treatment is an indication of the presence of rubella IgM. In point
number 3, if the antibody present is all maternal IgG, it will disappear from the infant's

circulation in 8 to 12 months. If, however,
antibody is of nonmaternal origin it will persist in the circulation.

g. Prevention. Obviously the best
method of prevention is to keep women in early
pregnancy away from cases of rubella. Since the
virus may be spread before the appearance of
clinical signs, this is often impossible. If a
known non-rubella immune pregnant woman is exposed and infected with rubella, the only possible method of prevention is by use of pooled
human gamma globulin (GG). The use of GG in
the case of rubella prevention has been a con-
troversial subject. A recent study using 0.5 cc
of GG per kg of body weight during a rubella
epidemic in a closed institution failed to show
any significant protective effect. Other workers
have reported various degrees of protection
ranging as high as 100 percent. The variation
in results is most likely due to: 1) time of
administration following exposure, 2) variation
in rubella antibody level of the GG, 3) the
dose of GG used. When studies were done using
a high antibody containing GG preparation at a
dose level of approximately 0.15 cc per lb of body
weight prior to rubella challenge, no cases were
induced. A preparation of this type, given intramuscularly at the above concentration within 6
days after exposure, appears to be the best
method of prevention available. In cases of lab-
oratory-verified rubella infection during pregnancy, the risks of possible fetal defects and
consideration of termination of pregnancy should
be discussed with the patient.

C.   DIAGNOSIS.
1. Clinical. Clinical diagnosis of postnatal rubella is made on the basis of location,
appearance and spread of the rash, along with
a history of exposure. In the absence of the
rash (rubella sine eruptione), a diagnosis is
impossible without laboratory studies.

2. *Laboratory*.
        a. <u>Virus Isolation</u>. In postnatal rubella,
the virus is present in the blood from 7 days
before until shortly after the rash appears.
The virus can be isolated from the pharynx from
one week before until a maximum of 14 days after
onset of the rash.   In the congenital rubella syndrome, the virus is present in the pharynx and
may be excreted in the urine for many months
after birth.   Virus isolation is carried out in
rabbit cornea or kidney or monkey kidney cell
lines or in primary human amnion or African green
monkey kidney (AGMK) cell cultures.   The cytopathic alterations produced by rubella virus are
not distinctive and, in the case of AGMK cells,
the virus must be detected by the interference
test using a known heterologous challenge virus
(see Chapter III).
        b. <u>Serology</u>. Rubella virus infection
induces the production of HI, CF and Nt antibodies
The HI test is most commonly used, but a fourfold
or greater increase in either HI, CF or Nt antibody titer between paired acute and convalescent
serums would be considered diagnostic.   Since the
CF antibodies appear and peak later than the HI
antibodies, the CF test may be useful in those
cases where the "acute" blood is collected several days after onset of rash and a diagnostic
rise in HI titer is not demonstrable.   The proper
interpretation of rubella serology is critical
in the assessment of congenital rubella.   The
demonstration of rubella virus specific IgM antibody (*e.g.*, by indirect immunofluorescence) would
be most helpful.   In congenital infection,
rubella IgM antibody persists in the mother as a
consequence of fetal infection.   As indicated
earlier, presence of rubella specific IgM antibody in the neonate would be considered diagnostic
The HI test is recommended as a screening test
for determination of rubella immunity.   An HI
antibody titer of 1:10 (or 1:8) or greater is considered indicative of rubella immunity.   Using

such a screening test, it is possible to determine
whether or not females in the child-bearing age
group are susceptible to rubella and to make
recommendations concerning vaccination.

D.   TREATMENT.
     1.   *Chemotherapy*. There is no available
chemotherapy for rubella. Treatment is symptomatic.

E.   EPIDEMIOLOGY.
     1.   *Transmission*. The virus is spread person
to person via the respiratory route by direct
contact. Except in the case of the rubella syndrome baby, carriers do not exist.
     2.   *Communicability*. The main source of the
spread of virus is the nasopharynx. Virus can
be demonstrated in the throat from 7 days before
until 7 days after the appearance of the rash.
Viremia occurs from 7 days before until the disappearance of the rash. The virus is also present
in urine and feces, but this source plays little
role in the spread of the disease.
     3.   *Characteristics of Epidemics*.
          a.   Seasonal Incidence. Rubella is endem-
ic worldwide, with the largest number of cases
occurring in late winter or early spring. Major
epidemics occur irregularly about every 9 to 10
years, with less extensive epidemics every 3 to
5 years. Widespread use of the rubella vaccine
will undoubtedly change this epidemic pattern.
          b.   Age. Most cases (40 percent) are
found in the age group from 5 to 9 years. Less
than 15 percent of the cases occur from age 0 to
5 years. Studies have shown that by age 20 to
25, 80 to 95 percent of the adult population
in the United States has rubella antibody by
virtue of natural contact.

F.   PREVENTION AND CONTROL.
     1.   *Artificial Passive Protection*. Gamma
globulin is used in the manner described under
"Congenital Rubella Syndrome."

    2. *Artificial* *Active* *Protection*. At the
present time there are three licensed rubella
vaccines. They are all similar in that they are
produced in tissue culture, contain live, attenuated virus, are given as a single subcutaneous
dose and give rise to about 95 percent rubella
antibody conversion. They differ in the strain
of virus used and the substrate on which the
virus is grown (canine kidney, duck embryo or
rabbit kidney cells). The antibody produced is
protective against natural rubella infection and
immunity has been shown to last at least 6 years.
Longer term protection is probable (perhaps
lifetime) but cannot be documented until more
time has elapsed following vaccine usage. Rash
and lymphadenopathy occasionally occur in children after vaccination, but small peripheral
joint pain is the most common complaint. Arthralgia or arthritis has been reported to occur in
1 to 15 percent of the vaccinated children. The
frequency and severity of joint pains are greater
in adult females, and in both cases begin 2 to
10 weeks after immunization and usually persist
for 1 to 3 days. Vaccinees shed virus for 1 to
4 weeks following vaccination, and, although
transmission to a susceptible contact is theo-
retically possible, the probability of vaccine
virus spread is exceedingly low. The vaccine
is recommended for all children between 1 year
and puberty. Priority should be given to
kindergarten and elementary school children.
Known non-rubella immune adolescent and adult
females are candidates for vaccination if pregnancy can be avoided for at least 2 months after
immunization. Contraindications for vaccine
use are: pregnancy, altered immune states,
severe febrile illness and hypersensitivity to
vaccine components.

G. CONTROL. Vaccination is the best method of
control. Isolation of known cases for at least
a week after the rash appears is helpful, but
since the period of contagiousness precedes the

clinical syndrome, this is not a highly successful method of control.   Nonimmune females during
gestation should be kept away from known or suspected rubella cases.

Part Four

ARBOVIRUSES

Chapter XXX

EASTERN EQUINE, WESTERN EQUINE, VENEZUELAN EQUINE, ST. LOUIS AND CALIFORNIA ENCEPHALITIS

There are more than 250 viruses which have been shown to be transmitted exclusively by the bite of an infected arthropod. About 80 of these have been shown to be capable of causing disease in humans. All are often referred to as arbo- viruses (arthropod borne viruses), a general grouping based on the method of transmission. The five viruses considered in this chapter are included in this broad classification, as is yel- low fever (Chapter XXXI). The large majority of the arboviruses are endemic in tropical areas and will not be considered in this text. However, in order to give some indication of the geograph- ical distribution and diversity of disease syn- dromes which they produce, a list of representa- tive members is given in Table 9.

A. PROPERTIES OF THE VIRUSES. Eastern, Western, Venezuelan and St. Louis Encephalitis (EEE, WEE, VEE and SLE) viruses have been biologically classified as members of the togavirus group. On the basis of common shared HI and CF antigens EEE, WEE and VEE are further serologically clas- sified as group A arboviruses. St. Louis enceph- alitis virus, by means of the same criteria, is classified along with yellow fever, Japanese B encephalitis, Dengue and several other viruses as a group B arbovirus. California encephalitis viruses and several other arboviruses appear to be distinct biologically and antigenically and are temporarily classified under the Bunyamwera supergroup. In all cases specific identification is made on the basis of neutralization. The toga- viruses contain single-stranded RNA as their ge- netic material, are enveloped, have a cubic icosa- hedral symmetry, and are 45 to 70 nm in size. They possess a hemagglutinin for red blood cells

TABLE 9   Clinical Syndromes Associated with Representative Arbovirus Infections

Clinical Manifestations	Arbovirus	Vector	Geographic Distribution
Encephalitis: *Prodromal* headache, chills and fever, nausea and vomiting, generalized pains and malaise; nuchal rigidity. Mental confusion, dysarthria, tremors, convulsions, and coma in severe cases; possible neurologic sequelae, especially WEE, EEE. Mild cases may show aseptic meningitis syndrome.	WEE (Gp.A)	*Culex* mosquito	Western USA, Canada.
	EEE (Gp.A)	*Aedes* mosquito	Eastern and Southern coastal USA.
	VEE (Gp.A)	*Aedes, Culex, Psorophora* mosquito	South and Central America, Southern USA.
	SLE (Gp.B)	*Culex* mosquito	Widespread in USA.
	JBE (Gp.B)	*Culex* mosquito	Far East (Japan, Korea, China, India).
	California group (Bunyamwera supergroup)	*Aedes* mosquito	North Central, Atlantic, and Southern USA; Trinidad, Brazil, Czechoslovakia, Yugoslavia, Mozambique.
Dengue (Breakbone) Fever: Headache, chills and fever, muscle and joint pain, maculopapular rash, lymphadenopathy.	Dengue (Gp.B): 4 serotypes	*Aedes* mosquito	Far East, Caribbean, Hawaii (tropics and subtropics).
Yellow Fever: Headache, chills and fever, backache, nausea and vomiting; jaundice, proteinuria, hemorrhage, leukopenia.	Yellow Fever (Gp.B)	*Aedes* mosquito	South America, Caribbean, Africa.
Hemorrhagic Fever: fever, petechiae or purpura, gastrointestinal, nasal, and uterine bleeding, hypotension, prostration, CNS signs, thrombocytopenia.	1. Tick-borne: RSSE (Gp.B)	*Ioxdes* ticks	Russia.
	2. Mosquito borne: Dengue, Yellow fever	*Aedes* mosquito	As previously designated.
	3. Enzootic: Lassa, Marburg, Tacaribe Gp. (Junin, Machupo)	Vector unconfirmed	Nigeria, Uganda, Argentina, Bolivia.
Mountain or Tick Fever, mild, febrile: chills, fever, headache, myalgia; ocular pain, joint and lumbar aches, nausea and vomiting, diphasic fever.	Colorado tick fever	*Dermacentor andersoni* tick	Pacific, Mountain areas of USA.
Undifferentiated Tropical Fevers: Headache, fever, malaise, myalgia, etc. (Dengue-like syndrome).	Gp.C (11 serotypes)	Mosquito-borne	Amazon, Panama, Trinidad.
	Sandfly fever group	*Phlebotomus* sandfly	Mediterranean, Russia, Asia, Central and South America.

Abbreviations Used: WEE, Western Equine Encephalitis; EEE, Eastern Equine Encephalitis; VEE, Venezuelan Equine Encephalitis; SLE, St. Louis Encephalitis; JBE, Japanese B Encephalitis; RSSE, Russian Spring-Summer Encephalitis.

from newborn chicks or geese. They are unstable
at room temperature but may be preserved in a
viable state for years when stored at -70°C in a
solution containing at least 10 to 25 percent protein (i.e., rabbit serum). They are readily inactivated by lipid solvents and sodium deoxycho-
late. They are formed in the cytoplasm of infected cells and acquire their membrane by "budding" from the cell surface.

B. HOST RESPONSE TO INFECTION.
    1. _Incubation Period, Signs and Symptoms_.
The incubation period is from 4 to 21 days. The
clinical picture with WEE, SLE, and VEE may consist of one of three types: 1) abrupt onset with
fever (105 to 106°F), nuchal rigidity, mental
confusion, speech difficulty, gastrointestinal
upset and occasionally spastic paralysis; 2)
prodromata of several days consisting of headache, fever and photophobia prior to the syndrome described above; 3) mild abortive cases
with low-grade fever and headache. Eastern
equine encephalitis infections usually run a
diphasic course consisting of a sudden onset with
fever, headache, and vomiting of 2 to 3 days
duration, a short period of well-being, and a
second phase with high fever, convulsions, drow-
siness and coma. Sequelae, which consist of
emotional instability or paralysis, may be seen
in up to 50 percent of those who survive. The
mortality may run as high as 70 percent. California encephalitis usually presents as a disease of abrupt onset with headache, fever which
may be as high as 104°F, vomiting and convulsions.
Sequelae are not often seen and the mortality is
very low.
    2. _Pathogenesis_. The virus enters the blood
stream by direct implantation from an infected
arthropod vector. It is removed from the blood
by the reticuloendothelial cells and multiplies
primarily in the spleen and lymph nodes, resulting in a secondary viremia. The central nervous
system is then invaded, probably by direct passage through the blood-brain barrier.

3. _Pathology_. In the case of St. Louis and
Western equine encephalitis similar central nervous system pathology is seen. The brain and
spinal cord show edema, vascular congestion and
small hemorrhages. There is a slight lymphocytic
infiltration of the meninges and widespread
lesions in the gray matter. The lesions consist
of focal glial cell accumulation, perivascular
lymphocytic infiltration (perivascular cuffing),
neuronal necrosis and ground substance degeneration. Eastern equine encephalitis cases show
generalized visceral congestion and pulmonary
edema. The central nervous system shows inflammation of the meninges, and lesions are most
obvious in the brain stem and basal ganglia.
There is destruction of neurons and ground substance and perivascular "cuffing." The spinal
cord is usually spared. In California encephalitis there is edema in the cerebral cortex,
perivascular "cuffing" and neuronal degeneration.

4. _Immune Response_. Neutralizing and hemagglutination inhibiting antibodies appear within
the first week after the onset of disease and
probably last for life. Complement fixing antibodies are detectable a short time later but
usually disappear within 2 years. Immunity to
the homologous virus probably lasts for life.

5. _Prognosis_. The prognosis in the case of
human infections with the viruses of Venezuelan
and California encephalitis is excellent. Convalescence may, however, be lengthy. Encephalitis
occurs in less than 3 percent of the clinical
cases and the mortality rate is below 0.5 percent. Western equine and St. Louis encephalitis
have a mortality rate of 2 to 10 percent, depending on the age of the patient and the epidemic.
St. Louis encephalitis is more severe in the
age group over 50 years with a mortality rate of
10 to 25 percent, and is less severe in children.
Western equine encephalitis is more severe in
children, where mortality may be high in certain
epidemics. Eastern equine encephalitis is a
severe disease especially in infants, where the

mortality rate may run as high as 70 percent.

In all of the arbovirus infections given above, the subclinical cases far outnumber the clinical ones. The ratio may be as high as 60 to 70 subclinical cases for every clinical one.

C. DIAGNOSIS.

   1. *Clinical*. A specific diagnosis cannot be made from the clinical signs and symptoms. Information as to whether or not the patient has recently been in an endemic or epidemic area can aid in diagnosis. The exact diagnosis must be made by laboratory tests.

   2. *Laboratory*.

      a. Isolation of the Virus. Virus isolation may be carried out by inoculation of susceptible tissue cultures such as hamster, African green or rhesus monkey kidney cells or by intracerebral inoculation into newborn mice or hamsters. The virus is present in the CSF, blood and nasopharynges in the acute stage of the disease. It is extremely difficult to isolate except in the first few days of illness. In fatal cases the virus may be recovered from the brain by the same techniques. Identification is carried out by serology.

      b. Serology. Three serological tests are applicable. They are complement fixation (CF), hemagglutination inhibition (HI) and neutralization (Nt). As with other serological tests they may be used to identify the virus isolate, or to indicate the presence of specific viral antibody. When paired serum specimens are used, the first specimen should be taken soon after the onset of the disease, and the second 2 to 3 weeks or later. The HI and CF tests primarily identify the virus group, while the Nt antibodies tend to be more type-specific. In all tests, the titer is highest against the homologous virus. A fourfold increase in titer between two successive serum samples is diagnostic.

D. TREATMENT. There is no specific treatment for the arbovirus encephalitides.

E. EPIDEMIOLOGY. Reservoirs of arboviruses
exist in a large number of mammals and birds.
In certain cases the virus has a very restricted
vertebrate-invertebrate cycle. The arthropod
acquires the infection while taking a blood meal
from an infected vertebrate and transmits the
disease through salivary secretions while taking
a second blood at a later time from a susceptible
host. The arthropod vector, though normal in
appearance, remains infected for life. In the
case of mosquitoes this is a matter of months.
The vertebrate usually recovers and eliminates
the virus. In the equine encephalitides,
horses may develop the disease, but, owing to the
short viremia, do not represent an important
reservoir for vector transmission, except in the
case of VEE. Man, in the case of the encephalitides discussed in this chapter, is an incidental
and "terminal" host. In the northern climate
it is possible that the virus survives the winter
by its presence in hibernating animals, reptiles,
or certain mosquitoes, or by existing over the
winter in a latent form in birds owing to their
temporary physiologic state. In the case of certain other arboviruses where the tick is the vector, there is a transovarial passage from one
tick generation to another. The main American
arbovirus encephalitides and their reservoirs
and vectors are given in Table 10. The diseases
are endemic throughout the year in tropical climates and occur mainly in late summer or early
fall in other areas. There are about 50 to 100
confirmed human cases of arbovirus encephalitis
reported annually throughout the United States.
The virus most frequently involved is SLE, with
a small number of infections due to EEE, WEE, CE
and VEE. Epidemics, which occur infrequently,
are usually confined to a limited geographical
area and are quickly brought under control. The
last epidemic in the United States was in south-
eastern Texas in 1971 and involved at least 63
humans and several thousand horses. The etiological agent in this outbreak was VEE.

**TABLE 10   Reservoir and Vector of the Most Common
American Arboviruses**

Arbovirus	Reservoir	Vector
WEE	Wild birds	*Culex tarsalis*
EEE	Wild birds	*Aedes, Culex* species
SLE	Wild birds	*Culex tarsalis* and *pipiens*
CE	Squirrels, rabbits, chipmunks	*Aedes* species
VEE	Wild birds	*Aedes, Psorophora* species

F. PREVENTION. There are no licensed vaccines
available for human use. There is a live attenuated virus vaccine against VEE available for use
in horses.

G. CONTROL. It is impractical to attempt to reduce or eradicate the vertebrate reservoir, but
highly practical to reduce the density of the
insect vector. This may be accomplished by spraying mosquito-infested areas with an insecticide
such as malathion. Since the viremia in the vertebrate host is short (3 to 6 days) a reduction
in the mosquito population will effectively break
the transmission cycle. Insect repellents and
mosquito netting aid in avoiding exposure in
endemic areas.

Chapter XXXI

YELLOW FEVER

A. PROPERTIES OF THE VIRUS. The virus of yellow fever is an arbovirus which contains single stranded RNA as its genetic material, is approximately 38 nm in size, is enveloped and has a capsid with cubic icosahedral symmetry. It is classified as a group B arbovirus in the togavirus group. Like most other arboviruses it possesses a hemagglutinin for goose or newborn chick red blood cells. It remains viable for several months when stored frozen in 50 percent glycerol, and is stable for years under the same conditions at -70°C. It is inactivated rapidly at 37°C and by lipid solvents or 0.1 percent formaldehyde. It is also inactivated by proteolytic enzymes such as papain or trypsin.

B. HOST RESPONSE TO INFECTION.
  1. _Incubation Period, Signs and Symptoms_.
The incubation period is from 2 to 6 days. The onset is sudden and marked by headache, chills, backache and fever which rarely exceeds 103°F. Nausea and vomiting are common. This syndrome, called the congestive stage, lasts 3 or 4 days and is followed by a drop in temperature. The period of stasis then sets in and the temperature rises but the pulse rate is slow relative to the fever (Faget's sign). Jaundice may occur, but in some cases is absent. In severe cases there are a marked albuminuria and hemorraghic manifestations. When death occurs it is usually 6 or 7 days after onset. Complications are infrequent and recovery is complete.
  2. _Pathogenesis_. The virus is implanted into a capillary beneath the skin by the bite of an infected mosquito. It spreads to the associated lymph nodes where it multiplies, a viremia ensues, and the virus localizes in the liver, kidney and spleen. It grows in these organs and causes extensive tissue damage.

3. _Pathology_. The main macroscopic findings in fatal cases of yellow fever are degeneration of the liver, kidney and heart. Jaundice is always present. Evidence of hemorrhage
is most often found in the mucosa at the pyloric
end of the stomach. The liver may also show
areas of hemorrhage. Microscopic examination
of the liver reveals widespread necrosis of the
cells in the midzonal area of the lobules.
There are less severely damaged cells adjacent
to the necrotic area and these cells show a
fatty degeneration consisting of small fat drop-
lets. The cytoplasm of the necrotic cells is
eosinophilic and shows areas of hyaline necrosis
(Councilman bodies). Nonspecific intranuclear
eosinophilic inclusions are also found in
hepatic cells.

4. _Immune Response_. Neutralizing antibodies
appear within the first week after the onset and
persist for life. Hemagglutinin inhibiting antibodies also rise early and are present for years
after infection. Complement fixing antibodies
appear after a variable period of time and disappear after 12 to 15 months.

5. _Prognosis_. Mortality may range from a
low of 5 percent to a high of 90 percent, depending upon the epidemic. Mild subclinical cases
occur. Among the signs and symptoms which carry
grave implications are early jaundice, prominent
albuminuria and cardiac involvement. There may
be extensive tissue damage but complete repair
takes place and there are no sequelae.

C. DIAGNOSIS.
1. _Clinical_. Any person, living in an endemic
yellow fever area and presenting with signs and
symptoms such as those given in I. B. 1., should be
suspected of having this disease. In an epidemic,
diagnosis of typical cases which follow the first
diagnosed case is not difficult. Cases which do
not follow a typical pattern can only be diagnosed
with the aid of the laboratory. Differential
diagnosis includes, malaria, viral hepatitis,
Leptospirosis icterohemorrhagica, and chemical or
drug toxicity.

2. *Laboratory*.
        a. Isolation of the Virus. The virus is
present in the blood from the onset of the disease for a period of 5 days. Blood serum suspected of containing the virus is inoculated by
the intracranial and intraperitoneal route into
newborn susceptible mice. It is advisable to
use two groups of mice, one which receives an
undiluted specimen and one a specimen diluted
1/10. The mice are examined daily for signs of
encephalitis and when such signs develop the
mice are killed, the brains harvested and ground
and the virus identified by the serological tests
given below. Postmortem, liver is the specimen
of choice.
        b. Serology. Three serological tests
are available. They are complement fixation
(CF), hemagglutinin inhibition (HI) and neutralization (Nt). In a primary infection with a
group B arbovirus such as yellow fever, the HI
and Nt antibodies appear early and are specific.
Subsequently heterologous group B, HI antibodies
appear and specificity is masked. The time of
appearance of CF antibodies is not consistent,
but when present they are specific. Any of these
tests which show a fourfold or greater increase
in antibody between serum specimens drawn in the
acute and convalescent stages of the disease are
diagnostic. The neutralization test is carried
out in mice and is therefore the most costly and
time-consuming. The diagnosis of yellow fever
(or any group B arbovirus) is difficult when the
infection takes place following a previous group
B infection. In this case there is a rapid rise
in heterologous HI, CF, and Nt antibodies which
masks the homologous antibody response.

D. TREATMENT. There is no specific treatment
for yellow fever. Special attention is paid to
bed rest, diet and rehydration.

E. EPIDEMIOLOGY. The disease is transmitted by
the bite of an infected mosquito. Two types of
disease cycle exist: the *urban*, where the

reservoir of infection is man, and the transmitting mosquito is a member of the Aedinae family, usually *Aedes aegypti*; and *jungle*, where
the reservoir of infection is monkeys and the
mosquito is a member of either the *Aedes* or
Haemogogus genus. Urban yellow fever often
exists in epidemics, but in jungle yellow fever,
man is a "chance" host. The virus must incubate
in the mosquito for about 2 weeks before transmission is possible, and mosquitoes remain infected for life. The disease is endemic in the
tropical areas of South or Central America,
Africa and the Caribbean.

F. PREVENTION. Effective active immunity
against yellow fever is produced by use of the
17D vaccine. It is a live virus preparation
which has been attenuated by passage in mouse and
fowl cells to a point where it is no longer
neurotropic or viscerotropic for man. The vaccine itself is prepared in chick embryos, lyophilized (freeze-dried) and rehydrated at time of use.
It is given as 0.5 ml subcutaneous inoculation
and produces immunity in 95 percent of the recipients. Immunity to infection has a duration of
at least 10 years. Reactions to the vaccine are
uncommon but, when present, consist of a mild
headache and fever which occur 5 to 15 days post-
inoculation. The vaccine is recommended for
persons over 6 months of age when living or
traveling in an endemic area, and for laboratory
personnel who might be exposed to the virus.
It is contraindicated in pregnancy, altered
immune states, steroid or antimetabolite therapy,
presence of severe underlying disease or sensitivity to chicken eggs.

G. CONTROL. Prevention of yellow fever outbreaks is best accomplished by breaking the transmission cycle. This may be accomplished by vaccination in man, and eradication of mosquitoes
by insecticide spraying. Further control is
brought about by requiring yellow fever vaccination of all individuals traveling to or from an
endemic area.

Part Five

UNCLASSIFIED DISEASES

Chapter XXXII

VIRAL HEPATITIS (SERUM HEPATITIS, INFECTIOUS HEPATITIS)

A. PROPERTIES OF THE INFECTIOUS AGENTS. There are a variety of viruses which can cause hepatitis in humans, but with the exception of yellow fever, it is an unusual manifestation of the disease. The term "viral hepatitis" is used for reference to two clinically similar syndromes, infectious (IH) and serum (SH) hepatitis. Until 10 years ago separation into either IH or SH was based upon the suspected method by which the patient acquired the disease, IH considered spread by the fecal-oral route, SH by parenteral inoculation with SH agent contaminated blood. The infectious agents associated with these syndromes have not been isolated and grown in the laboratory, but it seems unquestionable that the responsible agents are viral in nature. This conclusion has been reached after extensive serological, chemical, electron microscope, filtration and human to human transmission studies. For these reasons reference will be made to the agent of IH as the hepatitis A virus (HAV) and the agent of SH as hepatitis B virus (HBV). Similarly the diseases will be referred to as type A and type B hepatitis It must be remembered, however, that these "viruses" have not as yet been classified. The two syndromes are considered together so that they may be easily compared and contrasted.

1. *Hepatitis A Virus (HAV)*. The agent of infectious hepatitis (also referred to as type A or MS-1 hepatitis) has not been isolated in cell culture and has not been sufficiently characterized for inclusion in the physicochemical taxonomic scheme. Examination of stool filtrates from hepatitis A patients by immune electron microscopic techniques has revealed presence of spherical 27-nm virus-like particles closely resembling morphologically another unclassified agent, the Norwalk agent, the cause of some cases of

acute infectious nonbacterial gastroenteritis.
The size and appearance of these agents are
similar to members of the picornavirus or parvovirus (picodnavirus) groups. HAV is resistant to ether treatment, indicating absence of
essential structural lipids. Although the virus
can be destroyed by dry heat sterilization
(180°C for 1 hour), boiling (20 minutes), or
autoclaving (121°C at 15 pound pressure for
20 minutes), it is highly resistant to acid and
chemical disinfection. Empirically, 10 percent formaldehyde, 2 percent glutaraldehyde,
and ethylene oxide gas have been employed in
sterilization procedures because of their known
effectiveness against other viruses, including
some of the enteroviruses. A 0.5 percent to
1.0 percent sodium hypochlorite solution has
been found to be effective for disinfection of
water.

   2. _Hepatitis B Virus (HBV)_. Attempts to
cultivate the agent of type B (serum) hepatitis
in tissue culture have been unsuccessful. In
1964, Dr. Bernard Blumberg, while studying human
serum proteins by means of the agar double diffusion technique, detected an unusual antibody
in the serum of a hemophiliac. Hemophiliacs
require a large number of blood transfusions and
so it would be expected that antibodies would
be produced to a variety of antigens present in
the blood of the donors. The antibody reacted
with one serum specimen in a group of 24 from
"normal" persons. The serum against which it
reacted was from an Australian aborigine and so
the antigen was referred to as the Australia
(Au) antigen. At the outset, it was considered
to be a genetically determined serum protein,
but subsequent studies and astute observations
led to the conclusion that it was related to
type B (serum) hepatitis. It now appears that
the Au antigen represents the capsid of hepatitis
B virus. Thus it was referred to as the hepatitis
associated antigen (HAA) or Australia hepatitis
associated antigen (AuHAA).

HBV is very stable and is capable of surviving for over 6 months at room temperature and can be stored at -20°C for more than 20 years. Although relatively heat resistant (stable at 60°C for more than 1 hour), it is destroyed by dry heat sterilization (180°C for 1 hour), by boiling for 20 minutes, and by autoclaving at 121°C for 15 minutes. It is probably inactivated by 0.5 percent to 1.0 percent sodium hypochlorite. Empirical sterilization methods (10 percent formaldehyde, 2 percent glutaraldehyde, ethylene oxide) are similar to those employed for HAV. Ultraviolet irradiation of plasma or other blood products is ineffective in destroying HBV.

    a. <u>Nomenclature</u>. Three morphologic forms have been found in the serum of type B hepatitis patients by electron microscopic technique.

    1) A small, approximately 20 nm spherical particle, probably representing the viral coat or capsid of the virion. Ether treatment reduces its size, suggesting the presence of a lipid component.

    2) Filamentous forms.

    3) A complex sphere, 42 nm in diameter, consisting of a core and an outer surface component. This complex form has been termed the "Dane particle" after the investigator who first described it in 1970 and is believed to represent the virion *per se*. An enzyme called DNA polymerase which directs the synthesis of deoxyribonucleic acid has been found associated with the inner core of the Dane particle, providing indirect evidence that HBV may be a DNA virus. The surface component of the Dane particle is antigenically similar to the 20-nm particles and filamentous forms and manifests a group-specific antigenic determinant, <u>a</u>, and subtype-specific determinants, <u>d</u> or <u>y</u>, and <u>w</u> or <u>r</u>.

    b. <u>Revised Nomenclature</u>. The following revisions in nomenclature have been made by the Committee on Viral Hepatitis of the National Research Council-National Academy of Sciences.*

---

*Morbidity and Mortality Weekly Report: Volume 23, No. 4, for the week ending Jan. 26, 1974.

      1) HB_sAg--the hepatitis B antigen found on the surface of the Dane particle and on the unattached 20-nm particles.

      2) HB_cAg--the hepatitis B antigen found within the core of the Dane particle.

      3) Dane particle--a current term for the 42-nm particle containing HB_cAg in its core and HB_sAg on its surface.

      4) HBV--reserved for hepatitis B virus. The Dane particle may turn out to be HBV.

B. HOST RESPONSE TO INFECTION.
   1. *Clinical Picture*.
      a. Incubation Period. The presumptive mode of infection and the ensuing length of the incubation period have served in the past as differentiating features of type A (short-incubation) and type B (long-incubation) hepatitis.

Viral Hepatitis	Route of Infection	Incubation Period
Type A	Predominantly fecal-oral	2 to 6 weeks
Type B	Predominantly parenteral	6 to 26 weeks

      b. Signs and Symptoms.
      1) Prodromal--the preicteric stage is clinically difficult to distinguish and includes malaise, fatigue, anorexia, and gastrointestinal disturbances such as nausea, vomiting, and abdominal pain or discomfort. Arthralgia or nonmigratory symmetric polyarthritis may occur. Fever usually precedes icterus in hepatitis A and is less common in hepatitis B.

      2) Icteric stage--hepatomegaly and jaundice characteristically occurs in both types of hepatitis; however, anicteric cases are common. The icteric stage lasts for 1 to 3 weeks in hepatitis A and may be longer in hepatitis B.

     c. _Prognosis_.
     1) Hepatitis A--recovery is usually
complete and mortality rate is low (less than
1 percent). Possible development of chronic
active hepatitis has not been resolved.
     2) Hepatitis B--the clinical illness
is prolonged and usually more severe than in
hepatitis A. Although complete recovery occurs
in the majority of cases, case-fatality rates
have varied from 0.3 percent to as high as 36 percent. The severity and higher mortality of hepatitis B reflect in many cases underlying debil-
itating illnesses or conditions of patients who
contact the disease via blood transfusion.
Chronic active hepatitis may develop as a seque-
la of hepatitis B. A small proportion of
patients (2 to 10 percent) develop a chronic
carrier stage which may persist for years. It
is estimated that almost half of the HB_sAg (Au-HAA)
positive cases exhibit demonstrable evidence of
chronic liver disease on the basis of abnormal
liver function tests and histologic findings in
liver biopsy studies.
    2. Immune Response.
     a. _Hepatitis A_. Since specific immuno-
logic tests are not available for HAV, the exact
nature of the immune response has not been defined.
Patients develop high levels of IgM during the
acute stage of illness. Recovery is associated
with development of protective gamma globulin
antibody. Although the duration of immunity is
not known, it is apparently long-lasting.
Hepatitis A infection is most prevalent in children and young adults and there is widespread
resistance to reinfection in later adulthood.
There is no cross-immunity to hepatitis B infection.
     b. _Hepatitis B_. In natural hepatitis B
infection, the surface antigen (HB_sAg) appears
in the blood about 4 weeks prior to jaundice
and persists for about 4 to 5 weeks after onset
of the icteric stage. Serum IgM levels are
usually normal in anicteric cases, but may be
elevated in patients who develop jaundice.

Shortly after appearance of antigenemia, antibody against the core antigen (anti-HB$_c$) develops
before or at the time of serum transaminase elevation. The development of anti-HB$_c$, as detected
by the CF test, precedes appearance of antibody
against the surface antigen (anti-HB$_s$) by about
4 or more months. Anti-HB$_s$, as assayed by sensitive RIA and PHA methods, is detected about
2 months after antigenemia declines. In the
majority of cases of acute viral hepatitis B,
some degree of immunity to reinfection occurs.
The duration and subtype specificity of the
immunity have not been determined. No cross-
immunity develops against hepatitis-A infection.

The virus-host cell interaction is complicated by immunologic factors such as persistent
antigenemia, circulating antigen-antibody complexes, and impaired host response. If HB$_s$Ag
persists in the blood for more than 3 months
after onset of illness, the patient is likely
to become a chronic carrier and antigenemia is
demonstrable for many months to years. Anti-
HB$_c$ titers also persist at high levels in these
patients. The role of circulating antigen-antibody complexes in acute and chronic hepatitis
B has not been elucidated. Certain clinical
manifestations such as arthritis and arthralgias,
rash and urticaria, vasculitis, and hyperglobu-
linemia associated with hepatitis B may possibly
be immune in nature.

3. _Pathology_. The major clinical manifestations of the acute disease, either type A or B
hepatitis, stem from a functional failure due to
the degeneration of the parenchymal liver cells
or hepatocytes. Histopathologically, the diffuse parenchymal lesions are indistinguishable
in hepatitis A and B. Degenerative foci are
widely distributed within the architecturally
distorted hepatic lobules. Acidophilia and enlargement of the hepatocytes are evident and
Kupffer (reticuloendothelial) cells are predominantly found owing to hepatocyte necrosis.
Marked round cell infiltration is evident in the

portal areas. Bile stasis occurs as the parenchymal cells swell and block biliary excretion.
Hepatocyte regeneration usually occurs in 2 to
3 months. However, extensive hepatocellular
degeneration may lead to fibrosis and possible
post-necrotic cirrhosis.

C. DIAGNOSIS.
    1. *Clinical*. The physical findings are
similar in hepatitis A and B. Epidemiologic
history and length of the incubation period provide useful information for differential diagnosis of hepatitis A and B. Thus, those patients
presenting with jaundice and abnormal liver function tests and a history of blood transfusion or
parenteral inoculation within the past 60 to
180 days would be presumptively diagnosed as
having hepatitis B. Hepatitis A is usually associated with epidemics involving children and
young adults and has an abrupt onset of illness,
in contrast to the insidious nature of hepatitis
B, which affects all age groups.
    2. *Laboratory*.
        a. Liver Biopsy. Microscopic findings
on liver biopsy will confirm hepatic involvement
but will not differentiate hepatitis A and B.
        b. Biochemical Tests. Hepatic injury is
manifested by abnormal liver function tests.
Serum bilirubin, transaminase (SGOT, SGPT),
lactic dehydrogenase (LDH), and alkaline phos-
phatase levels are elevated. Thymol turbidity
usually rises to high levels in hepatitis A.
In hepatitis B, thymol turbidity is usually
normal in anicteric cases but may be markedly
increased in patients who develop jaundice. The
period to significant transaminase elevation is
relatively short in hepatitis A (3 to 19 days)
and prolonged in hepatitis B (35 to 200 days).
Transaminase levels which are normally below
50 units increase beyond 100 units and range
between 500 and 2000 units.
        c. Virologic Tests.
            1) Hepatitis A--specific virologic
tests are not available for HAV. The agent has

not been isolated in cell culture. Candidate
agents are currently being experimentally evaluated in marmoset monkeys.

      2) Hepatitis B--virologic tests
currently available are based on the immunologic
detection of hepatitis B surface antigen (HB_sAg)
or its homologous antibody (anti-HB_s). HBV has
not been isolated in culture, although it has
been experimentally transmitted to chimpanzees.

      a) Hepatitis B antigen--lab-
oratory confirmation of hepatitis B infection
and blood donor screening programs are based on
detection of HB_s antigenemia. HB_s antigenemia
is found in patients with acute and chronic type
B hepatitis and in asymptomatic carriers. In
acute hepatitis, HB_sAg is detected most frequently
early in the course of disease and may be undetectable by the third or fourth month during the
convalescent period. Owing to the transient antigenemia, a negative test for HB_sAg does not rule
out hepatitis B infection. Multiple sampling at
weekly intervals following onset of illness increases the frequency of HB_sAg detection.
Serologic methods recommended for HB_sAg detection on the basis of their sensitivity are radioimmunoassay (RIA) and passive hemagglutination
(PHA). However, most small hospitals presently
rely on counterimmunoelectrophoresis (CIEP),
even though its sensitivity is not as great. All
three tests are discussed in Chapter III.
Hepatitis B core antigen (HB_cAg) has not been
found in its free antigenic state in the blood
of hepatitis B patients. Immunofluorescent tests
have demonstrated its presence in infected
hepatocytes.

      b) Hepatitis B antibody--serologic
methods for determination of hepatitis B core
antibody (anti-HB_c), when they become generally
available, should provide an invaluable ancillary
tool for establishing HBV infection. Anti-HB_c
is a direct response to viral replication and
when measured by the CF test has been found in
all patients with active infection. In cases

where HB_sAg is not demonstrable because of its
transient nature, tests for anti-HB_c can be done
to establish current or recent infection. In
acute hepatitis, anti-HB_c appears early in the
course of illness before or at the time of serum
transaminase elevation. Anti-HB_c levels decline
following recovery but persist at high titers in
chronic HB_sAg carriers. In the case of anti-
HB_s, tests using RIA or PHA serve as important
serologic indicators for distinguishing primary
infection from reinfection. Because of its late
sequential development, anti-HB_s would not normally be detected in acute-phase blood. Its
appearance in convalescent-phase blood would
provide indirect evidence of HBV infection.
Anti-HB_s determinations also serve as epidemiologic markers for hepatitis B exposure in the
population.
                    c)   DNA polymerase activity--
hepatitis B specific DNA polymerase activity has
been demonstrated during the peak replication
period of HBV. Serum DNA polymerase activity has
been detected after HB_sAg appears in the blood
and before development of complement fixing core
antibody. The DNA polymerase activity has been
reported to persist for days or weeks in acute
cases and for months or years in chronic carriers.

D.   TREATMENT. Specific therapeutic drugs are
not available for hepatitis A and B. During the
acute stage of illness, the patient should get
adequate rest. Patients should abstain from
drinking alcohol because of its hepatotoxic
effects.

E.   EPIDEMIOLOGY.
     1.   _Transmission_.
          a.   Hepatitis A. Type A hepatitis is most
often spread by the ingestion of food and water
contaminated by feces from infected persons.
Explosive epidemics have occurred as a result of
sewage contamination of water supplies. Food-
borne outbreaks have also been associated with

the consumption of raw oysters or clams from HAV
sewage contaminated waters. Parenteral transmission via blood transfusion or the use of
contaminated needles and syringes is possible.
In the latter case, since the period of viremia
is short, the number of cases acquired by this
route is small. Sporadic cases and outbreaks
have occurred among individuals in close contact
with nonhuman primates, primarily chimpanzees.
A direct person-to-person spread by the respiratory route has not been demonstrated.

      b. <u>Hepatitis B.</u> Type B hepatitis is
transmitted primarily by infusion of blood or
blood products or through parenteral use of instruments (needles, syringes, tubing, etc.) contaminated with HBV. Cases occur sporadically,
with the highest incidence in those receiving
blood transfusions. The risk increases in proportion to the number of transfusions or units
of blood given. Outbreaks have occurred among
drug addicts owing to the use of needles and
syringes that were contaminated by HBV from the
blood of a carrier and subsequently used without
sterilization for parenteral inoculation of
another addict. Non-parenteral modes of transmission (oral and possibly venereal) have been
reported and are being investigated. Type B
hepatitis has also been transmitted by the oral
route experimentally in human volunteers.
Hepatitis B antigen has been found in stools and
urine of patients with this disease. Thus, it
is logical to assume that a low-grade fecal-oral
route of transmission is possible.

      2. <u>*Communicability*</u>.

      a. <u>Hepatitis A</u>. Feces from hepatitis A
patients have been shown to be infective 2 to 3
weeks prior to and 2 weeks following onset of
jaundice. However, it has been reported that
fecal excretion of HAV may continue for as long
as 1 year in some cases. Blood from these
patients is infective at least two weeks before
and less than 1 week following onset of icterus.

b.   Hepatitis B. Blood containing HB_sAg
is considered to be infective. HB_sAg has been
detected in blood from about four weeks preceding jaundice, and the antigenemia persists for
4 to 5 weeks or more following onset of the
icteric stage. The possible infectiousness of
stools and urine of acute hepatitis B patients
could be attributed to presence of blood in these
excreta. The extent of non-parenteral transmission (oral, venereal) by asymptomatic carriers
is not known. Hospital personnel and household
members in close contact with chronic-carrier
renal dialysis patients are at increased risk of
developing hepatitis B infection.
   3. Epidemiologic Features.
      a. Hepatitis A.
         1) Seasonal incidence--hepatitis A
is prevalent worldwide and occurs frequently as
either explosive epidemics or local outbreaks.
Common source epidemics attributed to contaminated water and food have occurred in the past
predominantly in the winter and spring months
but recent epidemiologic trends disclose a
greater seasonal variation in incidence. A distinct seasonal pattern has been reported in
shellfish-associated hepatitis, with a rise in
incidence in late autumn, a peak incidence in
winter, and a gradual decline in spring. Hepatitis related to ingestion of raw shellfish
usually occurs at a higher incidence in the
United States coastal states. Local outbreaks
of hepatitis A commonly occur in families and
institutions (schools, mental hospitals, prisons
and military installations) where there is close
personal contact. The fecal-oral route is the
main mode of transmission under these social
conditions.
         2) Morbidity--hepatitis A is pri-
marily an infection of children and young adults.
In children, the infection is usually mild, with
many abortive and subclinical infections.
Although the exact proportion of inapparent to
overt disease is not known, it is estimated that
the ratio of anicteric to icteric cases is at

least 10:1 in children. In adults, the disease
is more severe, particularly in women, and the
proportion of icteric cases is about equal that
of anicteric cases. Women developing hepatitis
during pregnancy or who are chronic carriers can
transmit the infection to their newborn infants.
Chimpanzee-associated hepatitis in animal
handlers is usually mild and is acquired during
close personal contact with infected animals.
Chimpanzees are believed to acquire the infection
from man.

     b.   Hepatitis B.

         1) Seasonal incidence--there are no
seasonal trends associated with hepatitis B, and
infections occur throughout the year. Hepatitis
B is worldwide in distribution and disease incidence varies according to geographic location.
Epidemiologic surveys have revealed that 1 to 5
per 1000 apparently healthy individuals in the
United States are HB_sAg "carriers."

         2) Morbidity--hepatitis B occurs
in all age groups. Children and old adults apparently acquire the infection predominantly via
blood transfusions (post-transfusion hepatitis).
Illicit drug use has contributed to a higher
incidence of hepatitis B in young adults, especially in metropolitan areas. The proportion of
anicteric to icteric cases has been estimated to
be more than 100:1. Health care personnel (medical, nursing, laboratory) are at greater risk
of acquiring infection due to direct contact
with hepatitis patients and HBV contaminated blood
specimens. Small outbreaks of hepatitis B have
occurred in hospitals, in some cases with no
history of parenteral inoculation or needle
exposure.

F.   PREVENTION.

    1. _Hepatitis A_.

      a. Artificial Passive Protection. Immune
serum globulin (adult gamma globulin) is reported
to prevent clinical illness in 80 to 90 percent

of exposed individuals when administered before
or within 1 to 2 weeks after exposure. ISG
reduces the severity of disease and does not
prevent infection. Therefore an active immunity
develops, in addition to the passive protection
afforded the individual. Under most conditions
of exposure, ISG is administered intramuscularly
at a dosage of 0.01 ml/lb body weight (approximately 0.02 ml/kg).

      b. <u>Artificial Active Protection</u>. A vac-
cine is not available against HAV.

    2. *Hepatitis B*.

      a. <u>Artificial Passive Protection</u>. Stan-
dard ISG employed for hepatitis A prophylaxis is
not effective against hepatitis B. A special
immune serum globulin preparation containing
high levels of anti-HB_s is being evaluated and
preliminary results are encouraging.

      b. <u>Artificial Active Protection</u>. No
vaccine is available at present against HBV.
In experimental studies with MS-2 strain HBV,
inoculation of heat-inactivated MS-2-containing
serum has been shown to confer protection
against subsequent challenge with HBV.

G. CONTROL.

    1. *Hepatitis A*. Control of hepatitis A
epidemics is based on sanitary measures to prevent fecal contamination of food and water
supplies. This includes a vigorous health
education program and constant monitoring of
sewage systems for efficiency of operation.
Possible carriers of HAV should be excluded
from food service handling and blood donation.
Hospitalized cases are kept in isolation and
instruments used for parenteral inoculation and
excreta are sterilized prior to disposal. Since
there are a large number of subclinical cases,
isolation *per se* cannot be a totally effective
control measure. Family members and others who
come into close contact with known cases are
often protected by the administration of gamma
globulin.

2. *Type B Hepatitis*. Hepatitis B$_s$ antigen
testing is now required on all blood to be used
for transfusion. Since the method most commonly
used for its detection (CIEP) is less than 100
percent effective, not all HBV-containing blood
will be discovered. A significant reduction in
the number of cases should, however, be effected.
As the efficiency of test methods improves and
the RIA and PHA systems are more widely used,
the number of type B hepatitis infections transmitted by blood transfusion should be further
reduced. There is also a distinct possibility
that there is a low-grade transmission of type B
hepatitis by the oral route, and for this reason
isolation of hospitalized cases is recommended.
Patients who have had hepatitis and known
asymptomatic chronic HB Ag carriers should not
be accepted as donors of blood for transfusion.
All instruments used parenterally in the management of patients who are known to have or suspected of having hepatitis should be sterilized.

Chapter XXXIII

MISCELLANEOUS DISEASES
WHICH MAY HAVE A VIRAL ETIOLOGY

A. CAT SCRATCH FEVER.
　　1. *Properties of the Infectious Agent*.
The etiological agent of this disease has not
been isolated. Attempts to grow the agent on
artificial media, tissue cultures, embryonated
eggs and in laboratory animals have been unsuccessful. It is possible that the infectious
agent is a member of the psittacosis-lymphogran-
uloma venereum group since the presence of
elementary bodies, similar to those seen in these
diseases, has been reported in stained sections
of infected lymph nodes.
　　2. *Host Response to Infection*.
　　　　a. Incubation Period, Signs and Symptoms.
The incubation period is 3 to 14 days. In about
half of the cases a lesion in the form of a small
pink papule appears at the site of a cat scratch
or bite. The lesion may be followed by an
adenitis of the regional lymph nodes which usually
lasts from 1 to 3 weeks. The inflammation is
occasionally accompanied by ocular (blepharitis,
follicular conjunctivitis), pharyngeal (acute
febrile sore throat) or neuromeningeal (encephalitis) signs. In certain cases a generalized
maculopapular rash may be present.
　　　　b. Prognosis. Most cases of the disease
are mild and resolve spontaneously in 1 to 3
weeks with complete recovery. Fatal cases, even
in encephalitis, have not been reported.
　　3. *Diagnosis*.
　　　　a. Laboratory Tests. Not routinely available.
　　　　b. Skin Test Reaction. Intradermal inoculation of a heat-inactivated antigen prepared
from pus from a lymph node of an infected case
will produce within 48 hours an erythematous
reaction (raised rose-colored papule a minimum
of 6 mm in diameter) in convalescent cat scratch

fever.   The reaction is highly specific.   The
antigen is not commercially available.

   4. _Treatment_.   There is no specific treatment.   It has been reported that tetracyclines
(adult dose 250 mg, 4 times a day for 8 to 10
days) shorten the course of the infection.

   5. _Epidemiology_.   The disease is worldwide
in distribution and occurs in all age groups.
The cat is the most common reservoir of the
infectious agent but does not itself become
overtly infected.   In most cases the disease
follows a cat scratch or bite, but it has been
reported to occur following thorn and plant
pricks and wood, metal and bone splinters.   It
is not uncommon to have epidemics within family
groups following close contact with a pet cat.
The extent of reinfection is not known.

   6. _Prevention_ _and_ _Control_.   There are no
specific methods of prevention or control.

B.   ERYTHEMA INFECTIOSUM (FIFTH DISEASE).   This
is a mild, exanthematous disease with cases
occurring mainly in children from 2 to 15 years
in age.   The incubation period is 5 to 14 days
and prodromal signs are usually absent.   A low-
grade fever may precede appearance of the rash.
The exanthem begins on the face as a flushing
and erythema of the cheeks ("slapped cheek appearance") and spreads to the trunk and limbs.
The maculopapular lesions have a characteristic
irregular reticular pattern as they fade and
coalesce.   They last for about 10 days and tend
to recur with exposure to sunlight or irritation
of the skin.   The etiologic agent is assumed to
be a virus and is probably spread by droplet
infection.   Epidemics occur in the early winter
or spring and affect girls more than boys.
Diagnostic laboratory tests are not available.
The prognosis is excellent and no specific therapy is recommended.

C.   EXANTHEM SUBITUM (ROSEOLA INFANTUM, SIXTH
DISEASE). This infection is one of the most
common eruptive fevers in young children, with
95 percent of the cases occurring between 6
months and 2 years of age. The incubation period
is 5 to 15 days and the clinical syndrome consists of fever, diarrhea and vomiting. The
fever, which may reach 105 to 106°F, has a rapid
onset, lasts for 3 to 5 days, and drops suddenly.
At this time a rash appears on the neck and trunk
but not the face and limbs. The eruption is
rubelliform in nature and usually disappears
within a day, and sometimes within hours, of its
appearance. The disease may occur without the
rash.

     Epidemics rarely occur and even within family
groups only one child will be infected. The
pathogenic agent is probably a virus but has not
been isolated. Its mode of transmission and
reservoir are not known. The disease is self-
resolving with complete recovery.

D.   GASTROENTERITIS. Epidemics of gastroenteritis which do not have a bacterial or known viral
(coxsackie, adenovirus, etc.) etiology have been
recognized for some time. The disease has a
rapid onset (1 to 2 days) and recovery (3 to 4
days). It is accompanied by a syndrome which
consists of mild systemic signs, abdominal pain
and diarrhea. In certain cases there are also
fever, chills and vomiting. The pathogenic
agent(s) has not been isolated but it is known
that the infection is highly communicable and is
worldwide in distribution. Candidate agents
include the Norwalk agent (possibly a parvovirus
or picornavirus), which produces an acute
abacterial gastroenteritis in all age groups, and
a reovirus-like agent associated with infant
diarrhea. These agents have been visualized by
the technique of immune electron microscopy, but
have not been isolated in laboratory animals or
in cell cultures. Treatment is symptomatic and
complete recovery is the rule.

GENERAL
REFERENCES

Behbehani, A.M.: Human Viral, Bedsonial, and
   Rickettsial Diseases: A Diagnostic Handbook
   for Physicians. Charles C Thomas, Spring-
   field, Illinois, 1972.

Bell, W.E., and McCormick, W.F.: Neurologic
   Infections in Children. W. B. Saunders,
   Philadelphia, 1975.

Davis, B.D., Dulbecco, R., Eisen, H.N.,
   Ginsberg, H.S., and Wood, W.B., Jr.: Micro-
   biology. Second Ed. Harper and Row,
   Hagerstown, Maryland, 1973.

Debré, R., and Celers, J.: Clinical Virology:
   The Evaluation and Management of Human Viral
   Infections. W. B. Saunders, Philadelphia, 1970.

Fenner, F.J., McAuslan, B.R., Mims, C.A.,
   Sambrook, J., and White, D.O.: The Biology
   of Animal Viruses. Second Ed. Academic
   Press, New York, 1974.

Fenner, F.J., and White, D.O.: Medical Virology.
   Academic Press, New York, 1970.

Hoeprich, P.D.: Infectious Diseases. Harper and
   Row, Hagerstown, Maryland, 1972.

Horsfall, F.L., and Tamm, I.: Viral and Rickettsial Infections of Man. Fourth Ed. J. B.
   Lippincott, Philadelphia, 1965.

Jawetz, E., Melnick, J.L., and Adelberg, E.A.:
   Review of Medical Microbiology. Lange,
   Los Altos, California, 1972.

Krugman, S., and Ward, R.: Infectious Diseases
of Children and Adults. Fifth Ed. C. V. Mosby,
St. Louis, 1973.

Kruse, P.F., Jr., and Patterson, M.K., Jr.:
Tissue Culture Methods and Applications.
Academic Press, New York, 1973.

Lennette, E.H., and Schmidt, N.J.: Diagnostic
Procedures for Viral and Rickettsial Diseases.
Fourth Ed. Am. Publ. Hlth. Assoc., New York,
1969.

Lennette, E.H., Spaulding, E.H., and Truant,
J.P.: Manual of Clinical Microbiology. Second
Ed. Am. Soc. Microbiology, Washington, D.C.,
1974.

Morbidity and Mortality Weekly Reports. U. S.
Department of Health, Education and Welfare,
Public Health Service. Published by the Center
for Disease Control, Atlanta, Georgia.

Wilner, B.I.: A Classification of the Major
Groups of Human and Other Animal Viruses. Fourth
Ed. Burgess, Minnesota, 1969.

Youmans, G.P., Paterson, P.Y., and Sommers, H.M.:
The Biologic and Clinical Basis of Infectious
Disease. W. B. Saunders, Philadelphia, 1975.

SELECTED
REFERENCES ▬▬▬▬

Classification of Animal Viruses (Chapter II)

Melnick, J.L.: Classification and nomenclature
  of animal viruses. Progr. Med. Virol.
  13:462-484, 1971.

_____: Classification and nomenclature of
  viruses. Progr. Med. Virol. 17:290-294, 1974.

Locather-Khorazo, D., and Seegal, B.C.: Intro-
  duction to viral ocular infections. *In* Microbiology of the Eye. C. V. Mosby, St. Louis,
  1972, pp. 267-277.

Fuccillo, D.A., Kurent, J.E., and Sever, J.L.:
  Slow virus diseases. Ann. Rev. Microbiol.
  28:231-264, 1974.

Isolation and Identification of Viruses (Chapter III)
and The Use of Acute and Convalescent Serum in
Viral Diagnosis (Chapter IV)

Gardner, P.S.: Rapid diagnostic techniques in
  clinical virology. *In* Modern Trends in Medical
  virology--2. Butterworths, London, 1970,
  pp. 15-50.

Sixth Annual ASCP Research Symposium: Laboratory
  diagnosis of viral infections. Am. J. Clin.
  Pathol. 57:731-847, 1972.

Hermann, E.C., Jr.: New concepts and developments
  in applied diagnostic virology. Progr. Med.
  Virol. 17:221-289, 1974.

Compromised Host Infections (Chapter V)

Seligmann, M., Fudenberg, H.H., and Good, R.A.:
  Editorial--A proposed classification of primary
  immunologic deficiencies. Am. J. Med.
  45:817-825, 1968.

Rosen, F.S.: The thymus gland and the immune
  deficiency syndromes. *In* Samter, M. (Ed.):
  Immunological Diseases. Vol. I. Second Ed.
  Little, Brown and Co., Boston, 1971, pp. 497-
  519.

Remington, J.S.: The compromised host. Hospital
  Practice, pp. 59-70, April 1972.

Antiviral Chemotherapy (Chapter VI)

Weinstein, L., and Chang, T-W.: Chemotherapy of
  viral infections. N. Engl. J. Med. 289:725-730
  1973.

Oncogenic Viruses (Chapter VII)

Gross, L.: Oncogenic viruses. Second Ed. Pergamon
  Press, New York, 1970.

Allen, D.W., and Cole, P.: Viruses and human cance:
  N. Engl. J. Med. 286:70-82, 1972.

Oncogenic Viruses (Chapter VII) Continued

Nakahara, W., Nishioka, K., Hirayama, T., and
Ito, Y.: Recent advances in tumor virology
and immunology. University Park Press,
Baltimore, 1972.

Tooze, J.: The molecular biology of tumor
viruses. Cold Spring Harbor Laboratory,
Cold Spring Harbor, New York, 1973.

Miller, G.: The oncogenicity of Epstein-Barr
virus. J. Infect. Dis. 130:187-205, 1974.

Adenoviruses (Chapter VIII)

Numazaki, Y., Shigeta, S., Kumasaka, T., Miyazawa,
T., Yamanaka, M., Yano, N., Takai, S., and
Ishida, N.: Acute hemorrhagic cystitis in
children. Isolation of adenovirus 11. N. Engl.
J. Med. 278:700-704, 1968.

Connor, J.D.: Evidence for an etiologic role of
adenoviral infection in pertussis syndrome.
N. Engl. J. Med. 283:390-394, 1970.

Mufson, M.A., Zollar, L.M., Mankad, V.N., and
Manalo, D.: Adenovirus infection in acute
hemorrhagic cystitis. A study in 25 children.
Am. J. Dis. Child. 121:281-285, 1971.

Center for Disease Control: Keratoconjunctivitis
due to adenovirus type 19--Canada. Morbidity
and Mortality Weekly Report 23 (No. 21): 185-186,
May 1974.

Cytomegalovirus (Chapter IX)

Hanshaw, J.B.: Congenital cytomegalovirus infection.
A fifteen-year perspective. J. Infect. Dis.
123:555-561, 1971.

Kantor, G.L., and Goldberg, L.S.: Cytomegalovirus-
induced postperfusion syndrome. Seminars in
Hematology 8:261-266, 1971.

Weller, T.H.: The cytomegalovirus: Ubiquitous
agents with protean manifestations. N. Engl.
J. Med. 285:203-214, 267-274, 1971.

Randall, J.L., and Plotkin, S.A.: Cytomegalovirus,
a model for herpesvirus opportunism. *In*
Prier, J.E., and Friedman, H. (Eds.): Opportunistic Pathogens. University Park Press,
Baltimore, 1974, pp. 261-280.

Herpes Simplex Virus (Chapter X)

Dudgeon, J.A.: Herpes simplex. *In* Heath, R.B.,
and Waterson, A.P. (Eds.): Modern Trends in
Medical Virology--2. Butterworths, London,
1970, pp. 78-115.

Nahmias, A.J., and Roizman, B.: Infection with
herpes simplex 1 and 2. N. Engl. J. Med.
289:667-674, 1973.

_____: Infection with herpes simplex 1 and 2.
Recurrent infection and cancer. N. Engl. J.
Med. 289:719-725, 1973.

Herpes Simplex Virus (Chapter X) Continued

_____: Infection with herpes simplex 1 and 2.
The infected host. N. Engl. J. Med. <u>289</u>:781-
789, 1973.

Infectious Mononucleosis (Chapter XI)

Henle, G., Henle, W., and Diehl, V.: Relation of
Burkitt's tumor-associated herpes-type virus
to infectious mononucleosis. Proc. Natl. Acad.
Sci. U. S. A. <u>59</u>:94-101, 1968.

Evans, A.S.: Infectious mononucleosis. Recent
developments. Gen. Pract. <u>40</u>:127-134, 1969.

Stites, D.P., and Leikola, J.: Infectious
mononucleosis. Seminars in Hematology
<u>8</u>:243-260, 1971.

Miller, G., Niederman, J.C., and Andrews, L.:
Prolonged oropharyngeal excretion of Epstein-
Barr virus after infectious mononucleosis.
N. Engl. J. Med. <u>288</u>:229-232, 1973.

Henle, W., and Henle, G.: Epstein-Barr virus and
infectious mononucleosis. N. Engl. J. Med.
<u>288</u>:263-264, 1973.

Influenza (Chapter XVIII)

World Health Organization Committee: A revised
system of nomenclature for influenza viruses.
Bull. W.H.O. <u>45</u>:119-124, 1971.

Influenza (Chapter XVIII) Continued

Eickhoff, T.C.: Immunization against influenza:
Rationale and recommendations. J. Infect. Dis.
123:446-454, 1971.

Kilbourne, E.D., Butler, W.T., and Rossen, R.D.:
Specific immunity in influenza--Summary of
influenza workshop III. J. Infect. Dis.
127:220-236, 1973.

Fox, J.P., and Kilbourne, E.D.: Epidemiology of
influenza--Summary of influenza workshop IV.
J. Infect. Dis. 128:361-386, 1973.

Kilbourne, E.D., Chanock, R.M., Choppin, P.W.,
Davenport, F.M., Fox, J.P., Gregg, M.B.,
Jackson, G.G., and Parkman, P.D.: Influenza
vaccines--Summary of influenza workshop V.
J. Infect. Dis. 129:750-771, 1974.

Center for Disease Control: Influenza surveillance:
Reye's syndrome and viral infections--United
States. Morbidity and Mortality Weekly Report.
23:58, February 1974.

Enteroviruses (Chapters XXIII, XXIV, and XXV)

Wenner, H.A.: The enteroviruses. Am. J. Clin.
Pathol. 57:751-761, 1972.

Rhinoviruses (Chapter XXVI)

Jackson, G.G., and Muldoon, R.L.: Viruses causing
   common respiratory infections in man.   I.
   Rhinoviruses.   J. Infect. Dis.   <u>127</u>:328-355, 1973.

Rabies (Chapter XXVIII)

Kaplan, M.M.: Epidemiology of rabies.   Nature
   <u>221</u>:421-425, 1969.

Plotkin, S.A., and Clark, H.F.: Prevention of
   rabies in man.   J. Infect. Dis.   <u>123</u>:227-240,
   1971.

Cox, H.R.: Rabies: Laboratory diagnosis and post-
   exposure treatment.   Am. J. Clin. Pathol.
   <u>57</u>:794-802, 1972.

Nagano, Y., and Davenport, F.M.: Rabies.
   University Park Press, Baltimore, 1972.

Rubella (Chapter XXIX)

Proceedings of the International Conference on
   Rubella Immunization.   Edit. by S. Krugman.
   Am. J. Dis. Child.   <u>118</u>:2-410, 1969.

Banatvala, J.E.: Rubella.   *In* Heath, R.B., and
   Waterson, A.P. (Eds.): Modern Trends in Medical
   Virology--2.   Butterworths, London, 1970,
   pp. 78-115.

Rubella (Chapter XXIX) Continued

Meyer, H.M., Jr., Parkman, P.D., and Hopps, H.E.:
The clinical application of laboratory diagnostic
procedures for rubella and measles (rubeola).
Am. J. Clin. Pathol. 57:803-813, 1972.

First Annual Symposium of the Eastern Pennsylvania
Branch, American Society for Microbiology:
Rubella. Edit. by H. Friedman and J. E. Prier.
Charles C Thomas, Springield, Illinois, 1973.

Arboviruses (Chapters XXX and XXXI)

Casals, J.: Arboviruses. Am. J. Clin. Pathol.
57:762-770, 1972.

Viral Hepatitis (Chapter XXXII)

Blumberg, B.S., Sutnick, A.I., London, W.T., and
Millman, I.: Australia antigen and hepatitis.
N. Engl. J. Med. 283:349-354, 1970.

Dane, D.S., Cameron, C.H., and Briggs, M.: Virus-
like particles in serum of patients with
Australia-antigen-associated hepatitis. Lancet
1:695-698, 1970.

Krugman, S., and Giles, J.P.: Viral hepatitis:
New light on an old disease. J.A.M.A.
212:1019-1029, 1970.

Viral Hepatitis (Chapter XXXII) Continued

Schulman, N.R.: Hepatitis-associated antigen.
Am. J. Med. 49:669-692, 1970

Feinstone, S.M., Kapikian, A.Z., and Purcell,
R.H.: Hepatitis A: Detection by immune electron
microscopy of a virus-like antigen associated
with acute illness. Science 182:1026-1028, 1973.

Krugman, S., Hoofnagle, J.H., Gerety, R.J.,
Kaplan, P.M., and Gerin, J.L.: Viral hepatitis
type B: DNA polymerase activity and antibody
to hepatitis B core antigen. N. Engl. J. Med.
290:1331-1335, 1974.

Hoofnagle, J.H., Gerety, R.J., Ni, L.Y., and
Barker, L.F.: Antibody to hepatitis B core
antigen. A sensitive indicator of hepatitis B
virus replication. N. Engl. J. Med. 290:1336-
1340, 1974.

Reed, W.D., Eddleston, A.L.W.F., and Williams, R.:
Immunopathology of viral hepatitis in man.
Progr. Med. Virol. 17:38-76, 1974.

Prince, A.M., Grady, G.F., Hazzi, C., Brotman, B.,
Kuhns, W.J., Levine, R.W., and Millian, S.J.:
Long-incubation post-transfusion hepatitis with-
out serological evidence of exposure to hepatitis-
B virus. Lancet 2:241-246, 1974.

Gastroenteritis (Chapter XXXIII)

Yow, M.D., Melnick, J.L., Blattner, R.J.,
Stephenson, W.B., Robinson, N.M., and
Burkhardt, M.A.: The association of viruses
and bacteria with infantile diarrhea. Am. J.
Epidemiol. 92:33-39, 1970.

Kapikian, A.Z., Wyatt, R.G., Dolin, R., Thornhill,
T.S., Kalica, A.R., and Chanock, R.M.: Visualization by immune electron microscopy of a 27-nm
particle associated with acute infectious non-
bacterial gastroenteritis. J. Virology
10:1075-1081, 1972.

Kapikian, A.Z., Kim, H.W., Wyatt, R.G., Rodriguez,
W.J., Ross, S., Cline, W.L., Parrott, R.H.,
and Chanock, R.M.: Reovirus-like agent in stools
Association with infantile diarrhea and development of serologic tests. Science 185:1049-1053,
1974.

VIRUS VACCINES

Disease	Substrate for Vaccine Production	Nature of the Vaccine	*Duration of Immunity	**Recommended Use	Booster Dose
Smallpox	Calf, sheep, chick embryo	Live attenuated	± 3 to 10 years	Risk groups only--no longer mandatory	Risk groups, every 3 years
Yellow fever	Chick embryo	Live attenuated	10 years, perhaps lifetime	High risk groups	High risk groups, every 10 years
Mumps	Chick embryo cell culture	Live attenuated	At least 6 years	All nonimmune 1 yr. old or over	None recommended
Influenza	Chick embryo	Inactivated	Very short (months)	Certain high risk groups	Re-vaccinate annually
Rabies	Duck embryo or rabbit brain	Inactivated	4 to 5 years	Certain conditions (usually postexposure)	Persons with continuing exposure every 2-3 years
Measles	Tissue culture (chick embryo, canine kidney)	Live attenuated	At least 8 to 10 years, perhaps lifetime	All nonimmune 1 yr. old or over	None recommended
Rubella	Tissue culture (canine kidney, rabbit kidney, duck embryo)	Live attenuated	At least 5 years, perhaps lifetime	All nonimmune 1 yr. old or over	None recommended
Poliomyelitis	Tissue culture monkey kidney, human lung	Live attenuated or inactivated	At least 5 years, perhaps lifetime	6-12 weeks of age, may be given to any age group	Booster dose upon entering school

*The exact duration of immunity is not known.

**See contraindications and recommendations under specific disease. Combined vaccines consisting of measles, mumps and rubella, measles and rubella or rubella and mumps have been licensed and proved effective and safe.

APPENDIX 2

BIOLOGICALS USED FOR PASSIVE IMMUNIZATION AGAINST VIRUS DISEASES

Disease	Source of Antiserum	Nature of Antiserum
Poliomyelitis	Human	Pooled immune serum globulin (ISG)* or poliomyelitis immune serum globulin.
Measles	Human	Measles immune globulin (MIG)** or pooled immune serum globulin (ISG)
Infectious hepatitis	Human	Pooled immune serum globulin (ISG)
Smallpox	Human	Vaccinia immune serum globulin (VIG)
Rabies	Equine	Hyperimmune horse antirabies serum
	Human	Human rabies immune globulin (HRIG) (obtained from volunteer vaccinees)
Varicella	Human	Zoster immune globulin (ZIG) (obtained from herpes zoster cases). (See recommendations, varicella.)

*The immune serum globulins (ISG) are sterile solutions, containing approximately 16.5 percent protein, obtained from large pools of human blood by cold alcohol fractionation.

**The specific disease immune serum globulins are obtained from volunteer vaccinees or convalescent cases of the given disease. In the case of equine antirabies hyperimmune serum, the horse is the "volunteer."

The effectiveness of passive immunization against rubella and mumps is questionable.

INDEX _____

Note: An overall list of virus names is pro-
vided under Infection (e.g., Infection, by
adenoviruses, by cytomegalovirus, etc.). For
detailed entries see also the specific viruses.

Acids, deoxyribonucle-
   ic in viruses 6,
   16
   nucleic, in viruses,
   6-7
   ribonucleic, in
   viruses, 6, 14-15
Acute respiratory
disease, 66-67
Adenovirus(es), detec-
   tion of, cyto-
   pathology in, 30
   hemagglutination
   in, 33
   inclusion bodies
   in, 31
   diseases caused by,
   ear, 23
   eye, 23
   gastrointestinal,
   25
   respiratory, 19
   salivary gland, 23
   urogenital, 26
   infection by, and
   acute respiratory
   disease, 66-67
   and conjunctivitis,
   67
   and epidemic kera-
   toconjunctivitis,
   67

and hemorrhagic
   cystitis, 67
and pertussis-like
   syndrome, 66-67
and pharyngocon-
   junctival fever,
   67
control of, 71
diagnosis of,
   clinical, 68-69
   laboratory, 69
epidemiology of,
   69-70
immune response
   to, 68
incubation period
   in, 66-67
pathogenesis of,
   67-68
pathology of, 68
prevention of, by
   active immuni-
   zation, 70
   by passive pro-
   tection, 70
prognosis in, 68
response of host
   to, 66-68
signs of, 66-67
symptoms of, 66-67

by herpesvirus, 30
by paramyxovirus,
   30
by picornavirus,
   29-30
by poxvirus, 30
Cytosar, in antiviral
   chemotherapy, 60
Cytosine arabinoside,
   in antiviral chemo-
   therapy, 60
Deoxyribonucleic acid-
   containing viruses,
   16
Detergents, effect of,
   on viruses, 12
Devil's grip, Cox-
   sackieviruses in, 150
Diagnosis, of infection,
      by adenovirus, 68-
      69
   by coronavirus, 118
   by Coxsackieviruses,
      152-153
   by cytomegalovirus,
      74-75
   by echovirus, 157-
      158
   by encephalitis
      viruses, 202
   by hepatitis A
      virus, 216
   by hepatitis B
      virus, 216, 217-
      218
   by herpes simplex
      virus, 81-82
   by measles virus,
      132-134
   by molluscum con-
      tagiosum virus,
      102
   by parainfluenza
      viruses, 142-143

by polioviruses,
   161-162
by rabies virus,
   174-176
by reoviruses,
   170-171
by respiratory
   syncytial vi-
   rus, 146-147
by rhinoviruses,
   167-168
by rubella virus,
   191-193
   in congenital
      rubella syn-
      drome, 190-
      191
by varicella-zoster,
   virus, 94-95
by variola virus,
   105-107
by virus causing
   infectious mono-
   nucleosis, 87-89
by virus causing
   lymphocytic
   choriomeningitis,
   115-116
by virus causing
   warts, 99-100
by yellow fever
   virus, 206-207
in compromised
   host, 55-56
serology in, 33-34,
   44-53. See also
   Test(s), sero-
   diagnostic.
Diffusion test(s), agar
   gel diffusion, 47
Diplornavirus, proper-
   ties of, chem-
   ical, 14
   physical, 14